CARLAT PSYCHIATRY

Psychiatry Practice Boosters, Third Edition

Edited by Thomas Jordan, MD, MPH

Published by Carlat Publishing, LLC
PO Box 626, Newburyport, MA 01950

Publisher and Editor-in-Chief: Daniel Carlat, MD
Executive Editor: Janice Jutras

This CME/CE activity is intended for psychiatrists, psychiatric nurses, psychologists, and other health care professionals with an interest in mental health. The Carlat CME Institute is accredited by the Accreditation Council for Continuing Medical Education to provide continuing medical education for physicians. Carlat CME Institute maintains responsibility for this program and its content. The American Board of Psychiatry and Neurology has reviewed *Psychiatry Practice Boosters* and has approved this program as a comprehensive Self-Assessment and CME Program, which is mandated by ABMS as a necessary component of maintenance of certification. Carlat CME Institute designates this enduring material educational activity for a maximum of four (4) ABPN Maintenance of Certification credits as part of the 2021 course. Physicians or psychologists should claim credit commensurate only with the extent of their participation in the activity. CME quizzes must be taken online at www.thecarlatreport.com.

Carlat Publishing books are available at special quantity discounts for bulk purchases as premiums, fund-raising, or for educational use. To order, visit www.thecarlatreport.com or call (866) 348-9279.

Print ISBN: 978-1-7329522-4-9
eBook ISBN: 978-1-7329522-5-6

1 2 3 4 5 6 7 8 9 10

Table of Contents

Acknowledgments

FOR THE THIRD EDITION of *Psychiatry Practice Boosters,* we have included even more reviews of research articles published in the past few years. The Carlat family of newsletters (*The Carlat Psychiatry Report, The Carlat Child Psychiatry Report,* and *The Carlat Addiction Treatment Report*) continues to grow along with the list of contributing authors. The original research updates adapted for this publication were authored by: Chris Aiken, MD, Bachaar Arnaout, MD, Rehan Aziz, MD, Stephanie Fenwick, PharmD, Brian Frankel, MD, Kristen Gardner, PharmD, Jessica Goren, PharmD, BCPP, Adrienne Grzenda, MD, PhD, Edmund S. Higgins, MD, Karen Hoffman, PhD, Thomas Jordan, MD, Jess Levy, MD, Xiaofan Li, MD, Donna Lisi, PharmD, Pavan Madan, MD, Jason Mallo, DO, Randall Moore, MD, Ahsan Nazeer, MD, Michael Posternak, MD, Xavier Preud'homme, MD, Nicholas Rosenlicht, MD, Adam Strassberg, MD, and Christian J. Teter, PharmD, BCPP. Special thanks to the editors reviewing the manuscript: Talia Puzantian, PharmD, BCPP, Chris Aiken, MD, Joshua Feder, MD, Benjamin Oldfield, MD, Osman Ali, MD, James Megna, MD, PhD, DFAPA, Brian McCarthy, MSN, PMHNP-BC, Peter Parry, MBBS, Jonathan Gamze, MD, Travis Lajoie, DO, and Janice Jutras.

Introduction

I F YOU ARE like most practitioners, you've probably developed a fairly standardized approach to treating patients. Over the years, it can become easy for your knowledge to stagnate. Yet, staying up to date with current literature is critical to providing good care. To help you keep track of recently published papers and avoid feeling overwhelmed, we've chosen recent journal articles that are most impactful for clinical practice. In addition, we've translated each article's statistical language into something easier to understand, allowing you to evaluate what change (if any) you should make to your practice.

The articles in this third edition of *Psychiatry Practice Boosters* are gleaned from the past two years of research updates in the Carlat family of newsletters. We include only a couple of the research updates published in the second edition, chosen because they are particularly helpful in clinical practice (eg, guidance on how to switch a patient from methadone to buprenorphine and the continued importance of lithium in psychiatric practice). The new updates address a wide range of topics on developments in psychopharmacology and psychotherapy, the increasing use of cannabis in the US, and studies relevant to the most common illnesses we treat in our daily practice.

HOW TO READ THESE UPDATES

We start by telling you where you can find the original study and what kind of study design it is. Refer to the introductory section on research design so that you'll better understand the jargon. The first paragraph of each update provides some context about the disorder or treatment being studied, and that's followed by a paragraph or two on the methodology of the study. We devote a paragraph to the results, followed by "The Carlat Take," which is our evaluation of the study's strengths or weaknesses—basically, this indicates whether we believe what the researchers have to say. Finally, we wrap up with "Practice Implications," a couple of lines telling you what, if anything, we think you should do differently in your practice as a result of the study findings.

Whether you should change your practice based on a single study is a matter of judgment, and you're welcome to disagree with our suggestions. Generally, if a clinical trial is very large and shows a marked advantage of a new treatment over placebo (or another treatment), there won't be a lot of debate—the treatment should find its way into your toolbox. But usually it's not so clear-cut. If a study is small, we only err on the side of recommending a new treatment if the intervention doesn't have a lot of risks, or if there simply aren't many options for the disorder in question. If the study is too small or its results are somehow problematic, we may take a wait-and-see approach.

A Quick Primer on Study Design and Statistics

RESEARCH ARTICLES ARE, by definition, chock-full of jargon describing research design and statistics. For those of you who need a quick refresher on this specialized vocabulary, here's a review of some of the most important topics.

HOW TO READ A RESEARCH ARTICLE

As you read a research article, you'll want to structure the information so that you can accurately absorb its essence as quickly as possible. Here's one approach you might find helpful. (This section was adapted from the article "How to Read a Journal Article," by Dr. Jeffrey Barkin, originally published in *TCPR*, Feb 2007.)

1. Who funded the study?

If a study is funded by a drug manufacturer, it is more likely to report results favorable to the sponsor's drug than studies funded by other sources (Lundh A et al, *Cochrane Database Syst Rev* 2012;12:MR000033). The reasons for this are not necessarily nefarious. Industry-funded studies are often very well designed, with large numbers of subjects and gold-standard research methods. One reason companies are more likely to get positive results is that they are careful about which drugs they choose to study. Often they will start with very small feasibility studies before deciding that a particular compound is worth the financial outlay for a large randomized trial. On the other hand, company-paid scientists sometimes engage in research trickery, such as setting up a control group for failure by providing a too-low dose of a comparison drug, or changing their statistical analyses after the fact to make their drug look better. While industry-funded studies can be valuable, you will need to give their conclusions more scrutiny than those funded by more objective sources, such as NIMH or private foundations. That said, not even NIMH researchers are completely free of bias—there's always an incentive to claim a positive result.

2. Are the patients being studied similar to the patients you treat?

Most randomized placebo-controlled trials have such strict inclusion criteria that their results may not apply to the patients in your office. For example, antidepressant trials often exclude patients with symptoms that are too mild or too severe, or patients with comorbid substance use, bipolar disorder, psychosis, or suicidality. One study concluded that patients who make it into research trials represent only about 20% of the patients whom real clinicians actually treat (Zimmerman M et al, *Am J Psychiatry* 2005;162(7):1370–1372).

3. What type of study design is it?

There's a hierarchy of medical evidence, from strongest to weakest. Later, I'll explain the different types of studies in more detail. But as an overview, the best evidence comes from **double-blind, randomized**

clinical trials. If such a trial includes a placebo group, it's even better. In **open randomized trials**, patients are randomized to treatments, but there is no attempt at blinding. Both the researchers and the patients are aware of the treatments, creating more opportunities for bias. Next on our list are **observational studies**, in which patients are not randomized to different groups, but rather are observed. There are many types of observational studies, and the terminology can get confusing.

A **cohort study** is a way of doing a controlled trial without having to assign subjects to groups. Here, two cohorts, or groups, are identified, one that received the treatment of interest and one that did not. Sometimes a cohort study is **prospective**, and sometimes it is **retrospective**. In a prospective cohort study, the two groups are observed prospectively (forward in time), studying the outcome under analysis for each group. A typical example of a prospective cohort study is a study of antidepressant use in pregnancy. Randomized trials are almost unheard of in pregnancy because of concerns about the possible risk to the fetus. Instead, researchers identify women with depression who happen to have been prescribed an antidepressant and compare them with a group with the same diagnosis who were not. Since the women were not randomized to the two groups, they may differ from one another in important ways. For example, women who opted to receive antidepressants may have been more depressed than the other group. If the study finds that infants exposed to antidepressants have more neonatal problems, it would therefore not be clear if the problems were caused by the medications or by the depression itself.

A **case series** is simply a description of a group of patients with a particular illness who have received a particular treatment. This is often retrospective, meaning that the author reviews old charts to extract information on a series of similar patients. Like open-label studies, these reports are suggestive but not definitive.

4. What are the identified primary and secondary outcomes of the study?

Studies are typically designed to assess a single primary outcome, such as percentage change in the Hamilton depression scale, rate of remission, or time to treatment discontinuation. These outcomes are generally chosen because they are the most clinically relevant measures. If the primary outcome does not reveal a difference between two groups, the authors will move on to a number of less relevant secondary outcome measures. There's nothing wrong with reporting secondary outcome measures—up to a point. Reporting too many extra outcomes can devolve into a statistical "fishing expedition," wherein a statistically significant difference is likely to appear by chance alone. The investigators may try to reel in that statistical noise with techniques like the Bonferroni correction, but these corrections are prone to errors of their own.

For this reason, savvy readers will focus on the results of predefined primary outcomes. Secondary results are meant to inform future research, not current practice.

5. How did the study deal with patients who dropped out?

Research patients drop out for various reasons, such as adverse events or clinical worsening, and there are different ways to account for these. The most conservative is called LOCF, or last observation carried forward. Here, each subject's last score is included, regardless of when the subject dropped out. As you can imagine, if an antidepressant causes many early dropouts, the LOCF method will tend to drag the final average depression score down, making the medication appear less effective. This is precisely the kind of information we need to know as clinicians, because the ideal medication should be both efficacious and well tolerated. By contrast, the weaker method of reporting results is called OC, or observed cases. Here, only the subjects who stayed in the study until the very end are counted, ignoring all dropouts. Somewhere between LOCF and OC is a complex statistical technique called MMRM, or mixed model repeated measures. Here, patients who dropped out are compared with similar patients who completed the study, and their scores are statistically extrapolated based on these comparisons.

6. Are the results both statistically and clinically significant?

In casual conversation, "significant" means big, but in research it simply means that the results are likely to be true, even if the results are very small. The larger the study, the more likely it is that the differences it measures are real. So when a study reports that one antidepressant has a "significantly" lower rate of nausea, look closely at the numbers. If the study is large enough, the results could be labeled significant even if the rates of nausea are 45% and 50% for the antidepressants being compared. Clinicians are interested in truth, but we also want to make a difference for our patients, and that's where we look to other measures like effect size and number needed to treat, which tell us how powerful a treatment really is. We get into more detail on these issues later in this section.

THE RANDOMIZED, PLACEBO-CONTROLLED, DOUBLE-BLIND STUDY: A DEEP DIVE

To begin with, let's decipher every researcher's favorite phrase: "A randomized, placebo-controlled, double-blind trial." This is sometimes abbreviated to "randomized controlled trial," or "RCT." The RCT is the gold standard of research studies, and many of our research updates summarize studies designed this way, so it's important that you understand exactly what the term means.

"Randomized"

If you want to fairly test whether one medication works better than placebo, or better than another medication, the patients chosen for the two study arms should be as equivalent as possible. Obviously, if the patients in the treatment group are much less depressed than those in the placebo group, a finding in favor of the antidepressant means very little. The easiest way to balance the two arms of a study is to randomly assign patients to one group or the other. In most papers, the authors will create a table comparing the baseline characteristics of the active group vs the placebo group, just to prove that their random assignment worked well—or to show that it didn't work so well after all.

"Placebo-controlled"

As clinicians, we see patients improve on medications all the time, but we are savvy enough to realize that many non-medication factors may be at play: positive expectation, changes in the patient's life, the natural course of the illness, the desire of patients to please you by saying they've improved even if they haven't, etc. All of these nonspecific factors come into play in research as well. A placebo control group allows us to measure the degree of nonspecific improvement vs medication improvement.

Uncontrolled studies and some open-label studies have neither a placebo control nor an active drug control. Generally, uncontrolled studies yield response rates that are much higher than those in controlled studies. Why is this so? After all, the presence or absence of a control group shouldn't affect the response rate of a completely separate group of patients who are given active treatment, should it? Oh, but it does, and the reason is that studies that include placebo groups are almost always (this is a teaser for the next paragraph) double blinded.

"DOUBLE-BLIND"

The purpose of a placebo group is to see how well patients do when they believe they are getting a particular treatment but are actually getting a sugar pill or some other nonspecific remedy. If they knew they were swallowing a placebo, they might very well still improve—from the passage of time, the attention of the research team, or other factors. But then a big part of the cure—the effects of the patient's faith in the prescription—would not be measured. So patients have to be fooled, and this is done by "blinding," a brutal term referring to the benign art of disguising the placebo pill as the active medication.

But keeping patients blind to the treatment is only one part of the story. The "double" in double-blind encompasses both the patient and the researcher. If a researcher knows that a particular patient is taking active medication, this knowledge may bias the evaluation of the patient's degree of improvement. Thus, double-blinding seeks to improve studies in two ways: first, by making the placebo group a more effective measure of nonspecific effects; and second, by reducing potential research bias.

Just as randomization can fail, leaving two unequal groups at the start of a trial, so can blinding. Subjects naturally try to figure out whether they got the placebo or the drug, and they are pretty good at guessing, especially if the drug is highly sedating. Investigators can check the integrity of the blind by asking the patients and their blinded physicians to guess which treatment they got, but this—unfortunately—is rarely done.

Another word for double-blind is "closed-label," in contrast with open-label studies where the patients know exactly what they're getting and researchers know exactly what they're dishing out. We've just said that open-label is not a great way of designing a clinical trial, so why are so many open-label studies published? Because they're much easier and cheaper to conduct. Nor are they devoid of value. Often an initial uncontrolled, open-label study identifies a drug as having promise for a given diagnosis, leading to a larger controlled study later on.

What about single-blind studies? Usually these are studies that compare two active drugs for a condition without including a placebo group. The patients know what they are taking. The doctor knows what the patients are getting. The only one who is blind is the rater, who is the one assessing the degree of clinical improvement using structured rating scales. This design still leaves plenty of room for the placebo to confound the results. Investigators might convey a tad more enthusiasm about one of those drugs to the subject, especially if the company that makes that drug is funding the study.

Non-pharmacologic trials. Placebos and blinding are relatively straightforward when testing medications. But what about non-pharmacologic clinical trials, such as studies on mindfulness therapy or internet-based CBT? In these cases, using a classic placebo control group is not an option. The control group can instead be set up with a different psychotherapy intervention, placement on a waitlist, or even a pharmacologic intervention that's already shown efficacy in the disorder being studied. Standardization of treatment intervention is very important, and the study will often mention the training of treatment providers or the use of manual-based therapies. Double-blinding the study is also a problem, as it's often impossible to blind the treatment provider or the patient receiving the therapy intervention, but single-blinding of the researcher administering the rating scales is standard practice.

STATISTICAL SIGNIFICANCE: WHAT DOES IT MEAN?

You won't get very far into any journal before you start reading about statistical significance and its close sibling, 95% confidence intervals (abbreviated as CI throughout this book). But what do these terms mean, and how do they help us draw conclusions about studies?

Let's say you are going old-school and doing a study comparing Prozac with placebo. Yes, it's been done before, but you want to make sure. Your primary outcome measure is the response rate, as measured by the trusty Hamilton depression scale. You find that 60 out of 100 people on Prozac responded vs only 40 out of 100 people on placebo. 60% is better than 40%, so you've once again proven that Prozac is an effective antidepressant, right? Not necessarily. It's possible that Prozac and placebo are equally effective, but that by pure chance 6 out of 10 people assigned to Prozac got better. An analogy is coin flipping. If you flipped a coin 10 times and got heads 6 times, would you automatically conclude that the coin is rigged—ie, that it is more effective at producing heads than tails? Probably not, because you'd expect that out of 10 coin tosses you might get more heads than tails or vice versa. But what if you tossed the coin 100 times? If you got 60 heads and 40 tails, you'd start to get suspicious that the coin is weighted toward heads. It's pretty unlikely that you'd get 60 heads by chance alone. Not impossible, mind you, but pretty unlikely.

Similarly, it's pretty unlikely, though not impossible, that you got a 60% response rate on Prozac by chance alone. The question that statistical significance aims to answer is, "Exactly how unlikely is it that this result is due to chance alone?" Let's say you do all your statistics and find that the difference between Prozac and placebo is statistically significant ($p = 0.03$). In this sentence, the "p" is for probability, meaning the probability that this difference occurred by chance alone (making it not a "real" finding) is 3 out of 100, or 0.03, or only 3%. The standard cutoff point for statistical significance is $p = 0.05$, or a 5% probability that the results occurred by chance, so you can feel confident calling your results significant.

You will often see studies in which results are reported like this: "The difference between Drug A and Drug B showed a trend toward statistical significance ($p = 0.06$)." This means that the results didn't quite meet the crucial 0.05 threshold, but they came close. Why is 5% the magic number? As befits an arbitrary number, its choice was also somewhat arbitrary. In 1926, R. A. Fisher, one of the fathers of modern statistics, wrote an article in which he argued that it was "convenient" to choose this cutoff point, for a variety of reasons related to standard deviations and the like (for more information, see Dallal GE, *The Little Handbook of Statistical Practice* at www.jerrydallal.com/LHSP/LHSP.HTM). This number has stood the test of time throughout all the scientific disciplines. Why? Because it has some intuitive appeal.

Look at it this way: Before we accept a finding as scientific fact, we want to be pretty certain that it didn't occur through some coincidence of random factors. But how certain is "pretty certain"? Would 80% certainty ($p = 0.2$) be enough for you? Probably not. Most doctors would not feel comfortable basing important treatment decisions on only an 80% certainty that a treatment is effective. Much better would be 99% certainty ($p = 0.01$), but if that were the required threshold, very few treatments would be shown as significantly better than placebo, and hence we would have very little to offer our patients. It just so happens that 95% certainty has felt right to scientists through the last 50 years or so. Of course it's arbitrary, but if we don't agree on some threshold, we open ourselves up to researchers creating their own threshold values depending on how strongly they want to push acceptance of their data (and some still do this anyway). Because the scientific community has settled upon $p = 0.05$, the term "statistical significance" has a certain, well, significance!

That being said, you, as a reader and clinician, have every right to look at a study reporting $p = 0.06$ and say to yourself, "There's only a 6/100 chance that this was a coincidental finding. It may not meet the 0.05 threshold, but at least in this clinical situation, that's good enough for me, so I think I'll try this treatment."

WHAT'S AN EFFECT SIZE?

Knowing that the apparent advantage of Prozac over placebo in these patients is statistically significant is all well and good. But how do we get a handle on measuring how strong this advantage is? This is where effect size comes into play. The effect size is the size of a statistically significant difference. To calculate it, you divide the difference between the two treatment groups' outcome measures by the standard deviation. (The standard deviation is how wide the data are spread out; in other words, how much overlap there is between the results of the treatment group and the placebo group.)

If the effect size is 0, this implies that the mean score for the treatment group was the same as the comparison group, ie, that there was no effect at all. And just as obviously, the higher the effect size, the stronger the effect of treatment. Here are the standard benchmarks: Effect sizes of 0 to 0.2 represent little to no effect, 0.2 to 0.5 a small effect, 0.5 to 0.8 a moderate effect, and 0.8 or greater a strong effect.

Here's an example of an effect size calculation. If the reduction in Hamilton depression score was 6.1 in the Prozac group and 4.4 in the placebo group, and the standard deviation was reported to be 3.9, the calculation for effect size would be: $(6.1 - 4.4) / 3.9 = 0.44$, which is just shy of a moderate effect size in favor of Prozac.

A moderate effect size is considered strong enough to be visible to the casual observer, so it might seem surprising that Prozac falls below that threshold. It's true. SSRIs consistently fall in the small effect range. But what that really means is that the difference between the SSRI and the placebo is too small for the casual observer to detect. The effect size removes the placebo effect, which for SSRIs accounts for about 1/3 of the benefits we see in practice.

Effect sizes for psychiatric treatments range from barely detectable (medications for generalized anxiety disorder are 0.3; PTSD medications are 0.2) to loud and clear (stimulants in ADHD are 0.7 to 0.8; exposure therapy for phobias is 1.0). Across all psychiatric treatments, from psychotherapy to

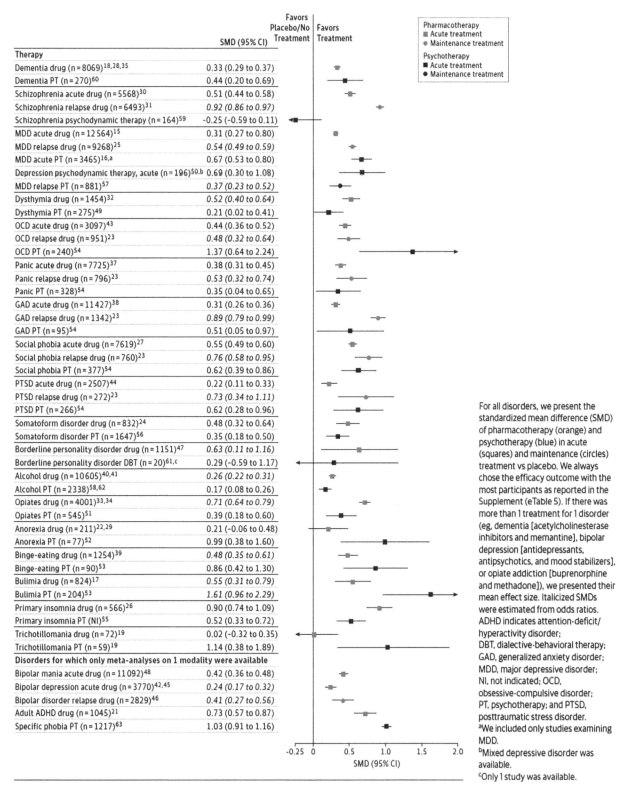

Therapy	SMD (95% CI)
Dementia drug (n = 8069)[18,28,35]	0.33 (0.29 to 0.37)
Dementia PT (n = 270)[60]	0.44 (0.20 to 0.69)
Schizophrenia acute drug (n = 5568)[30]	0.51 (0.44 to 0.58)
Schizophrenia relapse drug (n = 6493)[31]	0.92 (0.86 to 0.97)
Schizophrenia psychodynamic therapy (n = 164)[59]	-0.25 (-0.59 to 0.11)
MDD acute drug (n = 12 564)[15]	0.31 (0.27 to 0.80)
MDD relapse drug (n = 9268)[25]	0.54 (0.49 to 0.59)
MDD acute PT (n = 3465)[16,a]	0.67 (0.53 to 0.80)
Depression psychodynamic therapy, acute (n = 196)[50,b]	0.69 (0.30 to 1.08)
MDD relapse PT (n = 881)[57]	0.37 (0.23 to 0.52)
Dysthymia drug (n = 1454)[32]	0.52 (0.40 to 0.64)
Dysthymia PT (n = 275)[49]	0.21 (0.02 to 0.41)
OCD acute drug (n = 3097)[43]	0.44 (0.36 to 0.52)
OCD relapse drug (n = 951)[23]	0.48 (0.32 to 0.64)
OCD PT (n = 240)[54]	1.37 (0.64 to 2.24)
Panic acute drug (n = 7725)[37]	0.38 (0.31 to 0.45)
Panic relapse drug (n = 796)[23]	0.53 (0.32 to 0.74)
Panic PT (n = 328)[54]	0.35 (0.04 to 0.65)
GAD acute drug (n = 11 427)[38]	0.31 (0.26 to 0.36)
GAD relapse drug (n = 1342)[23]	0.89 (0.79 to 0.99)
GAD PT (n = 95)[54]	0.51 (0.05 to 0.97)
Social phobia acute drug (n = 7619)[27]	0.55 (0.49 to 0.60)
Social phobia relapse drug (n = 760)[23]	0.76 (0.58 to 0.95)
Social phobia PT (n = 377)[54]	0.62 (0.39 to 0.86)
PTSD acute drug (n = 2507)[44]	0.22 (0.11 to 0.33)
PTSD relapse drug (n = 272)[23]	0.73 (0.34 to 1.11)
PTSD PT (n = 266)[54]	0.62 (0.28 to 0.96)
Somatoform disorder drug (n = 832)[24]	0.48 (0.32 to 0.64)
Somatoform disorder PT (n = 1647)[56]	0.35 (0.18 to 0.50)
Borderline personality disorder drug (n = 1151)[47]	0.63 (0.11 to 1.16)
Borderline personality disorder DBT (n = 20)[61,c]	0.29 (-0.59 to 1.17)
Alcohol drug (n = 10 605)[40,41]	0.26 (0.22 to 0.31)
Alcohol PT (n = 2338)[58,62]	0.17 (0.08 to 0.26)
Opiates drug (n = 4001)[33,34]	0.71 (0.64 to 0.79)
Opiates PT (n = 545)[51]	0.39 (0.18 to 0.60)
Anorexia drug (n = 211)[22,29]	0.21 (-0.06 to 0.48)
Anorexia PT (n = 77)[52]	0.99 (0.38 to 1.60)
Binge-eating drug (n = 1254)[39]	0.48 (0.35 to 0.61)
Binge-eating PT (n = 90)[53]	0.86 (0.42 to 1.30)
Bulimia drug (n = 824)[17]	0.55 (0.31 to 0.79)
Bulimia PT (n = 204)[53]	1.61 (0.96 to 2.29)
Primary insomnia drug (n = 566)[26]	0.90 (0.74 to 1.09)
Primary insomnia PT (NI)[55]	0.52 (0.33 to 0.72)
Trichotillomania drug (n = 72)[19]	0.02 (-0.32 to 0.35)
Trichotillomania PT (n = 59)[19]	1.14 (0.38 to 1.89)
Disorders for which only meta-analyses on 1 modality were available	
Bipolar mania acute drug (n = 11 092)[48]	0.42 (0.36 to 0.48)
Bipolar depression acute drug (n = 3770)[42,45]	0.24 (0.17 to 0.32)
Bipolar disorder relapse drug (n = 2829)[46]	0.41 (0.27 to 0.56)
Adult ADHD drug (n = 1045)[21]	0.73 (0.57 to 0.87)
Specific phobia PT (n = 1217)[63]	1.03 (0.91 to 1.16)

For all disorders, we present the standardized mean difference (SMD) of pharmacotherapy (orange) and psychotherapy (blue) in acute (squares) and maintenance (circles) treatment vs placebo. We always chose the efficacy outcome with the most participants as reported in the Supplement (eTable 5). If there was more than 1 treatment for 1 disorder (eg, dementia [acetylcholinesterase inhibitors and memantine], bipolar depression [antidepressants, antipsychotics, and mood stabilizers], or opiate addiction [buprenorphine and methadone]), we presented their mean effect size. Italicized SMDs were estimated from odds ratios. ADHD indicates attention-deficit/hyperactivity disorder; DBT, dialectic-behavioral therapy; GAD, generalized anxiety disorder; MDD, major depressive disorder; NI, not indicated; OCD, obsessive-compulsive disorder; PT, psychotherapy; and PTSD, posttraumatic stress disorder.
[a] We included only studies examining MDD.
[b] Mixed depressive disorder was available.
[c] Only 1 study was available.

Source: Huhn M et al, *JAMA Psychiatry* 2014;71(6):706-715

medications, the average effect size weighs in at 0.5. That's fairly decent, but nothing to brag about. In general medicine, the average effect size is 0.45. See table on page 7 for examples of how effect sizes stack up across treatments.

BIBLIOGRAPHY

I've found two books to be extremely helpful in explaining research design. If you want to deepen your understanding of the topics I've touched on above, I suggest you read these.

Gehlbach SH. *Interpreting the Medical Literature.* 5th ed. New York, NY: McGraw-Hill Education / Medical; 2006.

Ghaemi SN. *A Clinician's Guide to Statistics and Epidemiology in Mental Health.* New York, NY: Cambridge University Press; 2009.

MOOD DISORDERS

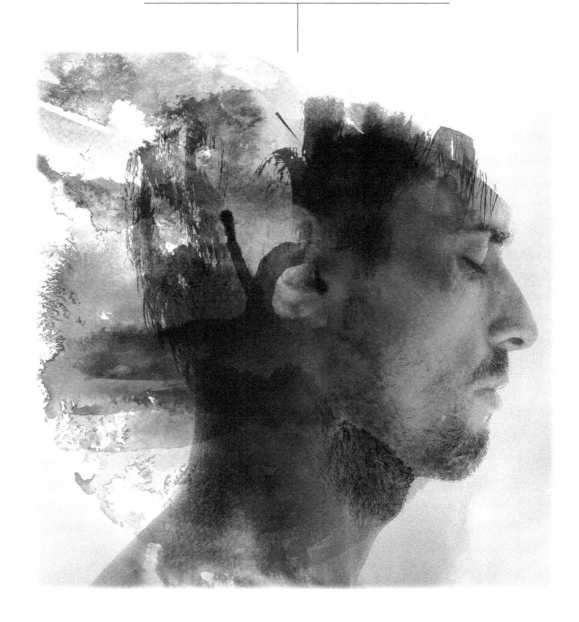

Does TMS Really Work in Depression?

REVIEW OF: **Yesavage JA, Fairchild JK, Mi Z, et al. Effect of repetitive transcranial magnetic stimulation on treatment-resistant major depression in US veterans: A randomized clinical trial.** *JAMA Psychiatry.* 2018 Sep 1;75(9):884–893.

STUDY TYPE: **Randomized, double-blind, sham-controlled trial**

REPETITIVE TRANSCRANIAL MAGNETIC stimulation (rTMS) has been FDA approved for treatment-resistant depression (TRD) since 2008. This non-invasive therapy uses an electromagnetic coil to stimulate electrical activity in the frontal cortex. The present study tested its efficacy in a Veterans Affairs (VA) population of TRD patients with complex comorbidities.

This was a double-blind, sham-controlled, randomized trial conducted across nine VA medical centers. In total, 164 subjects were enrolled; the average age was 55, and 81% were men. Treatment resistance was defined as 2 or more failed adequate antidepressant trials. Subjects had high rates of comorbidity, including PTSD (49%), medical comorbidity (49%), and a history of substance abuse (54%). Most were poorly functioning: Only 24% were working, and only 38% were married.

rTMS and sham rTMS were delivered for up to 30 sessions. Both groups came for treatment 5 days a week. Importantly, the sessions included supportive elements such as daily queries of mood and medication adherence and weekly screening for substance use. The primary outcome was remission of depression (≤ 10 on the Hamilton Depression Rating Scale).

RESULTS

rTMS displayed no advantage over sham treatment on the primary measure. Specifically, 41% achieved remission with active treatment, compared to 37% with sham treatment (p = 0.67). A sub-analysis suggested that rTMS might be more effective for depressed patients without comorbid PTSD (49% vs 43% remission rates), though this difference did not reach statistical significance either (p = 0.09). rTMS was very well tolerated.

THE CARLAT TAKE
Does this mean rTMS does not work? Not exactly, but it offered little benefit in this population of predominantly low-functioning men with complex comorbidities in the VA system. Remission rates were unusually high in both groups, and the fact that 40% recovered with sham treatment speaks to the therapeutic value of behavioral activation, structure, and social interaction in overcoming even the most seemingly refractory depressions.

PRACTICE IMPLICATIONS
When all the current research is considered, ECT is more effective than rTMS and should be the first-line treatment when depression has not responded to traditional pharmacotherapy (Chen JJ, *Behav Brain Res* 2017;320:30–36).

TMS: Deeper Is Not Better

REVIEW OF: Filipčić I, Filipčić IŠ, Milovac Ž, et al. Efficacy of repetitive transcranial magnetic stimulation using a figure-8-coil or an H1-coil in treatment of major depressive disorder: A randomized clinical trial. *J Psychiatr Res.* 2019 Jul;114:113–119.

STUDY TYPE: Randomized, single-blind, active-controlled trial

Seven transcranial magnetic stimulation (TMS) devices are FDA approved for depression, but only one—the Brainsway—is distinctly different from the others. Brainsway uses a patented H1 coil that penetrates deeper into the cortex than the standard figure-8 coil. Brainsway's marketing materials suggest that deeper is better, but the two versions of TMS have never been compared head to head—until now.

In this non-industry-sponsored study, 228 patients with moderate major depression were randomized to one of the following arms over 4 weeks: TMS with the H1 coil, TMS with the figure-8 coil, or 2 visits of standard psychopharmacology. All patients were taking an antidepressant and stayed on that medication during the trial. The evaluators were blinded, but the patients knew which treatment they were getting. The primary outcome was remission on the 17-item Hamilton Rating Scale for Depression (HAMD-17). The study was funded by a public psychiatric hospital in Croatia, which is where the treatments were conducted.

RESULTS

The H1 coil and figure-8 coil were not statistically different on the primary outcome of remission, although both were superior to the standard psychopharmacology group. On secondary measures, the H1 coil had a greater response rate on the HAMD-17 than the figure-8 coil, but there were no differences in the total change on the HAMD-17 or quality-of-life measures. Likewise, safety and tolerability were equal for both devices.

THE CARLAT TAKE
This is the first head-to-head study of the two rTMS devices, and its mixed results do not settle the score. Indirect comparisons of the two devices have been equally inconclusive, according to a meta-analysis of 19 trials (Gellersen HM and Kedzoir KK, *BMC Psych* 2019;19(1):139).

PRACTICE IMPLICATIONS
Despite company claims, deeper stimulation with the H1 coil does not work any better than earlier figure-8 coils.

Probiotics for Bipolar Disorder

REVIEW OF: **Dickerson F, Adamos M, Katsafanas E, et al. Adjunctive probiotic microorganisms to prevent rehospitalization in patients with acute mania: A randomized controlled trial.** *Bipolar Disord.* **2018 Nov;20(7):614–621.**

STUDY TYPE: **Randomized, double-blind, placebo-controlled trial**

PROBIOTICS, THE SO-CALLED "good" bacteria in the gut flora, have become popular as a natural treatment for various disorders. They are taken as capsules or through food sources like yogurt, vinegar, and fermented foods. Of relevance to psychiatry, some have theorized the existence of a "gut-brain axis," in which probiotics influence mood and behavior through the vagus nerve and the endocrine and immune systems. Probiotics have shown promise in small studies of anxiety, depression, cognition, and weight loss, and this trial tested whether a daily probiotic could lower the rate of rehospitalization after a manic episode.

The authors randomized 66 patients to receive either a probiotic or placebo as an adjunct to their usual medications after discharge from a hospital stay for mania. The probiotic capsule contained two bacterial strains that are found in breast milk and thought to modulate immune function: *Bifidobacterium lactis* BB-12 and *Lactobacillus rhamnosus* GG.

RESULTS

After 6 months, the number of patients with at least 1 rehospitalization was lower in the probiotic group (8 of 33, 24%) compared to those taking placebo (17 of 33, 51%). Three patients in the placebo group had more than 1 rehospitalization during the study period. However, the probiotic had no effect on manic and depressive symptoms (measured monthly using the Young Mania Rating Scale, Brief Psychiatric Rating Scale, and Montgomery–Åsberg Depression Rating Scale; YMRS, BPRS, and MADRS, respectively). No significant side effects were reported in this study.

THE CARLAT TAKE

It's interesting that the probiotic seemed to lead to such a stark reduction in rehospitalization rates, but did not improve patients' actual mood symptoms. Functional outcomes like hospitalization are arguably more important than symptom scales, but the lack of symptomatic improvement raises doubts about these results. A second randomized placebo-controlled trial of probiotics in bipolar disorder came out in 2020, and it noted only a non-significant trend in symptom reduction. If probiotics work in bipolar disorder, they must be addressing some aspect of the illness that isn't captured in our symptom rating scales (Shahrbabaki ME et al, *Iran J Psychiatry* 2020;15(1):10–16).

PRACTICE IMPLICATIONS

Probiotics have potential benefits for medical conditions that often accompany bipolar disorder, like metabolic and irritable bowel syndromes. On the other hand, they may not be safe for everyone. These "healthy bacteria" should be avoided in people who are pregnant, immu-nocompromised, or at high risk of infection, where probiotics pose known risks. The specific strains used in this study have a good safety record in humans, and they are available from online retailers as USANA-108 probiotic sticks and Culturelle Baby Grow + Thrive liquid.

Lithium Favored in Treatment Effectiveness Study

REVIEW OF: Lähteenvuo M, Tanskanen A, Taipale H, et al. Real-world effectiveness of pharmacologic treatments for the prevention of rehospitalization in a Finnish nationwide cohort of patients with bipolar disorder. *JAMA Psychiatry*. 2018 Apr 1;75(4):347–355.

STUDY TYPE: Retrospective cohort study

A NEW STUDY from Finland shows that lithium may be more effective than other treatments in reducing the risk of psychiatric rehospitalization in patients with bipolar disorder. Using a nationwide Finnish database, the authors examined the risk of rehospitalization for 18,000 patients with bipolar disorder—including psychiatric, cardiovascular, and all-cause rehospitalization—from January 1, 1987 to December 31, 2012, then determined the risk of a rehospitalization based on the patients' use of various medications.

RESULTS

Over the study period, 9,721 of the patients (54%) experienced at least 1 psychiatric rehospitalization. Patients on lithium had the lowest risk for all-cause rehospitalization (hazard ratio [HR] 0.71 [95% CI, 0.66–0.76]) and lithium had a robust effect for psychiatric rehospitalization (HR 0.67 [95% CI, 0.60–0.73]).

In addition to the findings on lithium, researchers also revealed the following about other psychotropic treatments:

- Long-acting injectable formulations of antipsychotic medications were more effective than their oral antipsychotic counterparts at reducing the risk of psychiatric rehospitalization (HR 0.70 [95% CI, 0.55–0.90]).
- Quetiapine fumarate, the most frequently used antipsychotic treatment in the population, was only modestly effective at reducing the risk of psychiatric rehospitalization (HR 0.92 [95% CI, 0.85–0.98]).
- Benzodiazepines were linked to an increased risk for both psychiatric and all-cause rehospitalization (HR 1.19 [95% CI, 1.12–1.26]).

THE CARLAT TAKE

Although most of our treatment guidelines are based on randomized controlled trials, observational studies have many important findings to contribute to evidence-based medicine, and they are an alternative means to gauge effectiveness of various treatments.

PRACTICE IMPLICATIONS

The study findings correlate well with our clinical and anecdotal experience. Lithium is highly effective for bipolar disorder and should be a first-line treatment; it is also particularly effective for maintenance therapy. Long-acting injectable antipsychotics may be more effective than their corresponding oral agents in preventing rehospitalizations, and we should consider their use whenever feasible. Long-term benzodiazepine use remains risky and problematic.

Suicide Rates in College Students

REVIEW OF: **Mortier P, Auerbach RP, Alonso J, et al. Suicidal thoughts and behaviors among first-year college students: Results from the WMH-ICS project.** *J Am Acad Child Adolesc Psychiatry.* **2018 Apr;57(4):263–273.e1.**

STUDY TYPE: **Cross-sectional study**

ADOLESCENCE IS A time of high risk for suicidal thoughts and behaviors (STB), and rates are rising. In those ages 15–29, suicide is the second leading cause of death globally (www.who.int/mental_health/prevention/suicide/suicideprevent/en). A recent article published some interesting survey data, giving us a clearer picture of how common STB is and what some of its causes are. Full-time, freshman college students at 19 colleges in eight countries were surveyed.

RESULTS

The response rate was 45.5%, and the final sample included 13,984 responses (54% female; mean age 19). Approximately one-third of all respondents reported STB at some point during their lifetime. The median age of onset of STB was 14, with 75% of cases starting before age 16. More than half of those with ideation at some point in their life transitioned to a suicide plan, and a quarter of planners attempted suicide.

The strongest correlate for STB and transition from ideation to attempts was non-heterosexual orientation, yet it was notable that students who identified as heterosexual but with same-sex attraction also had a significantly elevated risk of transitioning from suicidal ideation to development of a plan.

THE CARLAT TAKE

Suicidal ideation and behavior are distressingly common among first-year college students worldwide. The transition to adulthood and self-differentiation makes this a particularly vulnerable period. Those with non-heterosexual orientation may be at even higher risk.

PRACTICE IMPLICATIONS

This study tells us to double down on screening our own patients and pressing for more screening efforts. In addition, prevention initiatives and gatekeeper training are effective in decreasing suicidality and increasing help-seeking. Where resources are limited, campus outreach could specifically target high-risk first-year students.

Resilience Networks in Adolescent Females at Risk for Major Depression

REVIEW OF: Fischer AS, Camacho MC, Ho TC, Whitfield-Gabrieli S, Gotlib IH. Neural markers of resilience in adolescent females at familial risk for major depressive disorder. *JAMA Psychiatry*. 2018 May 1;75(5):493–502.

STUDY TYPE: **Prospective cohort study**

ONE OF OUR biggest in-office challenges is how to enhance teen resilience, the process of adapting to and recovering from stressful life experiences. Some neuroscientists hypothesize that resilience is related to the limbic system, which plays a vital role in emotion processing, motivation, and learning. According to one theory, when people can exert better modulation of the limbic system, they are at lower risk of depression. A group of researchers recently looked at these neural pathways in adolescent females, and there were some intriguing results.

Fischer and colleagues examined brain pathways of resilience in adolescent females at familial risk for depression. They conducted a longitudinal study at Stanford University from 2003 to 2017. Sixty-five subjects participated: 20 at high risk of MDD in whom depression did not develop (resilient), 20 at high risk in whom depression developed (converted), and 25 at low risk of MDD with no history of psychopathology (control). Outcomes measured via functional MRI scans included connectivity in the limbic, salience, and executive control networks. Participants were imaged once, on average at age 19, 6 years after beginning the study.

RESULTS

The researchers found that resilient adolescent females had greater connectivity between the limbic and executive control systems than did subjects who developed depression or even controls. The strength of the connection was correlated with positive life events.

THE CARLAT TAKE

This study is consistent with the hypothesis that high-risk but resilient adolescent females have greater executive system control over emotions and behavior arising from the limbic system, which perhaps insulates them against depression.

PRACTICE IMPLICATIONS

What are the treatment implications of this small study? Theoretically, since positive life events were correlated with better neural resilience, we might want to focus on therapeutic approaches that have an activity-oriented style and are designed to strengthen adaptive coping and cognitions, thereby helping teens foster positive life experiences.

Optimal Antidepressant Doses in Major Depression

REVIEW OF: Furukawa TA, Cipriani A, Cowen PJ, et al. Optimal dose of selective serotonin reuptake inhibitors, venlafaxine, and mirtazapine in major depression: A systematic review and dose-response meta-analysis. *Lancet Psychiatry.* 2019 Jul;6(7):601–609.

STUDY TYPE: Systematic review and meta-analysis

MOST ANTIDEPRESSANTS DO not have a linear response curve. In other words, the benefits level off as the dose goes up. If the dose gets too high, the side effects start to outweigh those diminishing returns. What's not clear is where the "sweet spot" lies for each antidepressant, and this study set out to capture that optimal dose range.

This dose-response meta-analysis included 77 double-blind, randomized, placebo-controlled trials of fixed-dose SSRIs (except fluvoxamine), venlafaxine, and mirtazapine in major depression (n = 19,365). Median trial length was 8 weeks (range = 4–12 weeks). Primary outcomes were efficacy (treatment response defined as 50% or greater reduction in depressive symptoms), tolerability (dropouts due to adverse effects), and acceptability (dropouts for any reason).

TABLE: **Antidepressant Dosages**

ANTIDEPRESSANT	OPTIMAL DAILY DOSE
Citalopram	20–40 mg
Escitalopram	10–15 mg
Fluoxetine	20–40 mg
Mirtazapine	15–30 mg
Paroxetine	20–30 mg
Sertraline	50–100 mg
Venlafaxine	75–150 mg

From the Article: "Optimal Antidepressant Doses in Major Depression" *The Carlat Psychiatry Report*, Volume 18, Number 3, March 2020 www.thecarlatreport.com

RESULTS

The best balance of efficacy, tolerability, and acceptability was achieved at low to medium doses of these antidepressants (see table and graph). At higher doses (> 40 mg of fluoxetine equivalents), the benefits plateaued and dropouts from side effects showed steep, linear-to-exponential curves. Venlafaxine was unique in that its efficacy continued to increase up to 375 mg, though it started slowing at doses above 150 mg.

THE CARLAT TAKE

These results show that the low to medium range of antidepressant doses may be most appropriate for patients with depression. It's often helpful to keep charts like this close by when considering a change in medication. After this publication, a second study appeared using the same data but stratified by age. That analysis clarified that the elderly—those over age 60—were particularly vulnerable to the adverse effects of higher doses of antidepressants (Holper L, *EClinicalMedicine* 2020;18:100219).

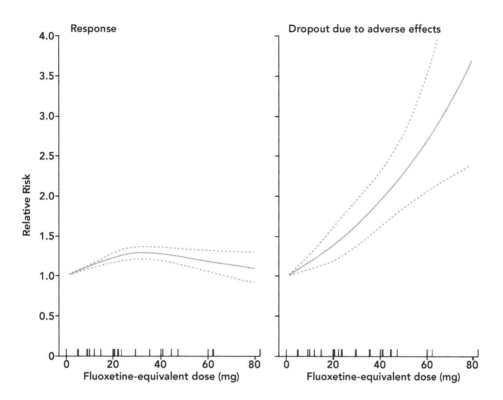

GRAPH: Relationship of Dose to Response and Adverse Effects for SSRIs Across 99 Treatment Groups (Furukawa TA et al, 2019).

From the Article: "Optimal Antidepressant Doses in Major Depression" *The Carlat Psychiatry Report*, Volume 18, Number 3, March 2020 www.thecarlatreport.com

PRACTICE IMPLICATIONS

When a patient does not recover fully on an antidepressant, it's tempting to keep raising the dose. That strategy may work sometimes, but this study suggests that for many on second-generation antidepressants, an increased dose is more likely to cause side effects than therapeutic gains, particularly for those over age 60. If you go to a higher dose, measure the outcomes, and consider dropping back down if there's no clear improvement.

PSYCHOSIS MANAGEMENT

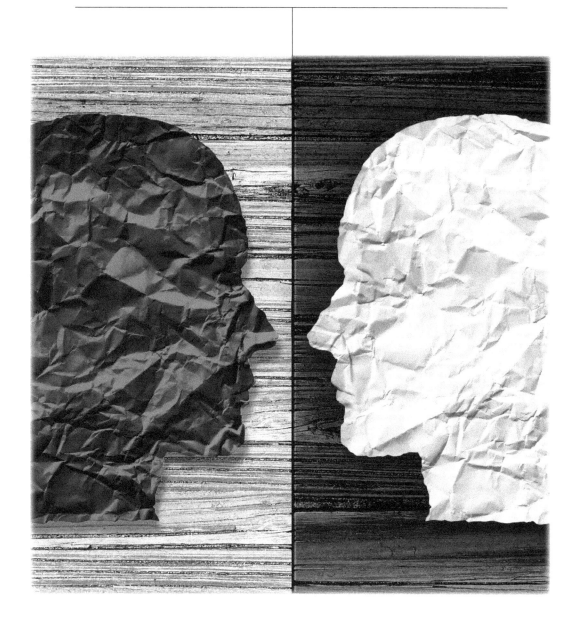

Cannabidiol for Schizophrenia

REVIEW OF: McGuire P, Robson P, Cubala WJ, et al. Cannabidiol (CBD) as an adjunctive therapy in schizophrenia: A multicenter randomized controlled trial. *Am J Psychiatry*. 2018 Mar 1;175(3):225–231.

STUDY TYPE: Randomized, double-blind, placebo-controlled trial

TRADITIONAL ANTIPSYCHOTIC MEDICATIONS leave much to be desired. Their therapeutic response rate for schizophrenia is low, and their side effects are troubling and lead to high rates of noncompliance. Clearly, there is an urgent need for alternative agents. Although patients—including those diagnosed with schizophrenia—have long attested to the benefits of marijuana, only recently have researchers begun taking it seriously as a therapeutic option. In this pilot study, investigators evaluated the benefits of cannabidiol (CBD), which is one of the two main active components of marijuana (the other being tetrahydrocannabinol or THC), for the treatment of schizophrenia.

In this 6-week trial, adult patients diagnosed with schizophrenia or a related psychotic disorder were recruited from sites across Europe. All patients were actively psychotic, though they could not be entirely treatment-resistant (ie, patients had to have displayed at least a partial response to antipsychotic medications). Patients entered the study only after they had been on a stable dosage of antipsychotic medication for at least 4 weeks, and this medication was continued throughout the course of the study. 43 patients were randomized to CBD and 45 to placebo. CBD was dosed at 1,000 mg/day in the form of an oral solution. Active substance use was not grounds for exclusion. The primary efficacy measure used was the Positive and Negative Syndrome Scale (PANSS), while cognition was measured using the Brief Assessment of Cognition in Schizophrenia (BACS) scale.

RESULTS

Positive symptoms (eg, delusions or hallucinations) were significantly reduced at the 6-week endpoint for patients receiving CBD compared to placebo. Improvement in negative symptoms (eg, flat affect) favored CBD, but this difference did not reach statistical significance. Patients receiving CBD also fared better on global assessment of functioning, clinicians' global assessment of improvement, and cognitive measures, though this latter difference fell just short of statistical significance ($p = 0.07$). No major adverse events occurred that were attributed to CBD, and the participants were not able to tell if they were taking CBD or placebo.

THE CARLAT TAKE

CBD's therapeutic potential has received a lot of attention lately. This is the most rigorous study of CBD in schizophrenia to date, and its intriguing findings warrant replication with a larger sample and longer duration. The dose of 1,000 mg/day is also important to recognize. A similar study published a few months later showed no significant effect of CBD at a dose of 600 mg/day for positive or negative symptoms associated with schizophrenia (Boggs DL et al, *Psychopharmacology* 2018;235(7):1923–1932).

PRACTICE IMPLICATIONS

Given the many limitations and pitfalls associated with traditional antipsychotic medications, a novel compound that might be devoid of those pitfalls is a most welcome development. Currently the only prescription CBD product is Epidiolex, which is FDA approved for some forms of childhood epilepsy, though it must be used with caution due to potent induction of multiple CYP450 enzymes. Over-the-counter CBD products can vary widely in quality and may contain THC as well. The current research into medicinal CBD and THC products also varies; in a recent systematic review the dose of CBD ranged between 2.5 and 1,000 mg/day (Sarris J et al, *BMC Psychiatry* 2020;20(1):24). Right now the research is too early for us to recommend a particular product or dose schedule of CBD for treatment of psychiatric disorders.

Is Clozapine the Next Step After a Single Failed Antipsychotic Trial?

REVIEW OF: **Kahn RS, van Rossum IW, Leucht S, et al. Amisulpride and olanzapine followed by open-label treatment with clozapine in first-episode schizophrenia and schizophreniform disorder (OPTiMiSE): A three-phase switching study.** *Lancet Psychiatry*. 2018 Oct;5(10):797–807.

STUDY TYPE: **Sequential trial with open-label and randomized, double-blind comparison phases**

CLOZAPINE IS OFTEN used as a last resort in schizophrenia, even though practice guidelines recommend a trial of this medication after failing 2 antipsychotics. The current study set out to test a treatment algorithm based on those guidelines in patients with first-episode psychosis.

Researchers recruited a total of 446 patients from 27 clinics in various European countries. All patients were in their first psychotic episode and had diagnoses of schizophrenia (51%), schizophreniform disorder (43%), or schizoaffective disorder (6%). To refresh your memory, schizophreniform disorder means that symptoms of schizophrenia have been present for more than a month but less than 6 months. The average age was 26; most were male (70%) and Caucasian (87%). The primary outcome was symptomatic remission on the Positive and Negative Syndrome Scale (PANSS). The trial was funded by the European Commission.

The patients were entered into a three-phase study:

▥ Phase 1: All 446 patients were prescribed open-label amisulpride, an antipsychotic used outside the US for schizophrenia but approved by the FDA in 2020 for postoperative nausea and vomiting (as Barhemsys injection), for 4 weeks at ≤ 800 mg/day.
▥ Phase 2: Those patients who did not achieve remission on amisulpride were randomly assigned to a double-blind trial of either continuing amisulpride or switching to olanzapine (≤ 20 mg/day, mean 16 mg/day) for 6 weeks.
▥ Phase 3: Patients who did not respond to either amisulpride or olanzapine were treated with open-label clozapine (≤ 900 mg/day, mean 490 mg/day) for 12 weeks.

Amisulpride and olanzapine were selected for this algorithm because their effect sizes are second only to clozapine's in schizophrenia.

RESULTS

Just over half (56%) of the patients remitted during the first phase of antipsychotic treatment with amisulpride. Of the 93 patients who started the second phase, about 32% remitted with either amisulpride continuation or olanzapine switch, with no significant differences between these drugs. Finally, 40 patients were left to assign to clozapine; 18 of those completed the 12-week trial, and 5 (28%) achieved remission.

THE CARLAT TAKE

Because switching to olanzapine did not yield better outcomes than continuing the first antipsychotic, the authors suggested that this second-line switch could be skipped and that patients who don't respond to their first antipsychotic might be better served by going straight to clozapine. Studies have continued to support the use of clozapine in severely ill patients despite its significant risks for metabolic syndrome, weight gain, and Type 2 diabetes (Masuda T et al, *JAMA Psychiatry* 2019;76(10):1052–1062).

PRACTICE IMPLICATIONS

Moving clozapine up from step 3 to step 2 in the schizophrenia algorithm is a bold suggestion. We'd like to see that tested out in a more controlled manner before changing practice guidelines. What these results do tell us is that schizophrenia recovery can take time. If patients haven't recovered after 10 weeks, whether with one antipsychotic or two, a trial of clozapine is not unreasonable, but it's not clearly the best option either.

Dose Maintenance or Reduction With Antipsychotics?

REVIEW OF: Zhou Y, Li G, Li D, Cui H, Ning Y. Dose reduction of risperidone and olanzapine can improve cognitive function and negative symptoms in stable schizophrenic patients: A single-blinded, 52-week, randomized controlled study. *J Psychopharmacol.* 2018 May;32(5):524–532.

STUDY TYPE: Randomized, single-blind, active-controlled trial

ONCE PATIENTS WITH schizophrenia are stabilized on an antipsychotic in the acute phase of their treatment, guidelines are unclear on how to continue dosing. Some guidelines recommend lowering the dose, others recommend maintaining the dose, and others give no firm recommendations whatsoever. For fear of relapse, many clinicians never lower the dose, so many patients are simply kept on the higher acute-phase doses. These doses can be associated with more side effects, including extrapyramidal symptoms, metabolic syndrome, and impaired cognitive function.

This 52-week, single-blinded (rater-blinded), randomized controlled study sought data on maintenance and reduction using two frequently prescribed antipsychotics. Relapse was defined as a score of ≥ 4 on the Positive and Negative Syndrome Scale (PANSS) on at least one of the following: delusions, conceptual disorganization, hallucinatory behavior, or suspiciousness.

Researchers studied 75 stabilized schizophrenic patients, who were prescribed either risperidone (≥ 4 mg/day) or olanzapine (≥ 10 mg/day). They were randomly divided into a maintenance group (n = 38) and a dose-reduction group (n = 37). In the maintenance group, the dose of medication remained unchanged. In the dose-reduction group, the dose of antipsychotic was reduced by 25% for the first 4 weeks, then reduced by 50% of the original dose for the remaining 48 weeks. Doses were never lowered below minimum recommendations—ie, below 2 mg/day for risperidone or below 5 mg/day for olanzapine.

RESULTS

Over 52 weeks, relapse rates were not significantly different between the groups, with relapse of only 4 patients in the dose-reduction group and 6 patients in the maintenance group. A 50% dose reduction of antipsychotics did not lead to any worsening of psychotic symptoms. In fact, patients on the lower doses had fewer extrapyramidal symptoms ($p = 0.012$), lower body mass index ($p = 0.005$), improved cognitive function ($p = 0.001$), and improved negative symptoms overall ($p < 0.001$).

THE CARLAT TAKE

It's important to note that this research supports dose reduction, not elimination, of antipsychotic medication for stable patients. Despite a small sample size, using single rather than double blinding, and being limited to only two antipsychotics, this study offers much-needed evidence to guide some important clinical decisions.

PRACTICE IMPLICATIONS

During the maintenance phase for our stabilized patients with schizophrenia, careful antipsychotic dose reduction (by 25% over the first 4 weeks, and then by 50% thereafter) is worth trying. The improvement in side effects and cognitive functioning may be well worth it to our patients.

Steroid-Induced Psychosis in the Pediatric Population

REVIEW OF: **Hodgins GE, Saltz SB, Gibbs EP, et al. Steroid-induced psychosis in the pediatric population: A new case and review of the literature.** *J Child Adolesc Psychopharmacol.* **2018 Jun;28(5):354–359.**

STUDY TYPE: **Case report and literature review**

CHILDHOOD PSYCHOSIS IS a rare disorder, and accurate diagnosis is crucial. Recently, clinicians at the University of Miami Miller School of Medicine reported a case of steroid-induced psychosis in a pediatric patient.

In the case report, a 12-year-old Haitian girl was diagnosed with discoid lupus erythematosus after she presented with fever, fatigue, and anemia. She was started on prednisolone and hydroxychloroquine, and a few days later presented with mutism, drooling, and altered mental status. She was admitted to the PICU, and her symptoms were assumed to be related to her lupus; therefore, she was treated with IV prednisolone. After eight days of admission, the patient remained disoriented, mute, and paranoid. After a negative organic workup, the psychiatry consultation team recommended tapering the steroid and started her on clonazepam 0.25 mg BID and risperidone 0.5 mg BID (later switched to haloperidol). After 12 days, the patient was much improved—she was more verbal and had no hallucinations. Once the steroid was entirely discontinued, she became completely organized and was discharged on haloperidol 5 mg/day and lorazepam 1 mg twice daily.

RESULTS

The authors did a literature review and found 15 other case reports of steroid-induced psychosis in children and adolescents. Asthma was the most common indication for the initiation of steroids. The higher the dose of steroids (> 40–80 mg dose equivalents per day), the more chances of psychiatric manifestations.

THE CARLAT TAKE

This case highlights the need to search for specific causes of psychotic symptoms that can usually be resolved, avoiding unnecessary long-term treatments. Especially in young children, primary psychotic disorders are rare, and any psychotic symptoms should prompt a thorough search for a secondary reason.

PRACTICE IMPLICATIONS

For steroid-induced psychosis, discontinuation of steroids is the gold standard and typically completely resolves the symptoms within a few days to a month. For instances where steroid taper is not possible, a trial of benzodiazepines and antipsychotics can be helpful.

Weight Gain From Aripiprazole Same as Risperidone

REVIEW OF: Schoemakers RJ, van Kesteren C, van Rosmalen J, et al. No differences in weight gain between risperidone and aripiprazole in children and adolescents after 12 months. *J Child Adolesc Psychopharmacol.* 2019 Apr;29(3):192–196.

STUDY TYPE: Retrospective cohort study

MANY PROVIDERS PREFER aripiprazole over risperidone for young patients due to observed lower incidence of weight gain. This is supported in studies with follow-up of less than 3 months. However, does aripiprazole fare better with long-term use?

Researchers reviewed records of children and adolescents treated with aripiprazole or risperidone for at least 12 months at a Dutch mental health organization between 2008 and 2015. Only 89 of 874 patients on risperidone and 42 on aripiprazole met the inclusion criteria, as over 80% of the charts had missing baseline and/or follow-up data.

RESULTS

BMI z-scores (age- and sex-adjusted BMI) significantly increased for both medications over 12 months. The increase was marginally lower for aripiprazole (0.30, 95% CI = 0.07–0.53) than for risperidone (0.37, 95% CI = 0.21–0.53), but not statistically significant (p = 0.97). Of note, the aripiprazole group had a higher BMI z-score at baseline (0.18) compared to the risperidone group (−0.33), possibly as aripiprazole is preferred over risperidone for overweight kids.

The authors predicted that an 11-year-old boy with a BMI of 16.9 at baseline would have a predicted BMI of 18.2 with aripiprazole use for 12 months and 18.4 with risperidone, whereas that same boy would have a BMI of 17.5 without medications for that year.

THE CARLAT TAKE

In this study, using aripiprazole to avoid weight gain was fruitless, at least in children. Children are much more vulnerable to metabolic side effects than adults, so we can't apply these discouraging results to all patients. The small sample size dampens our confidence in the results, but BMI z-scores offer a more accurate understanding of weight gain.

PRACTICE IMPLICATIONS

If we must use antipsychotics in children, "old-school" measures like packing lunch for school and eating dinner with the family, plus reducing fast food and screen time, can have an enormous positive impact on a child's physical and mental well-being. Periodic assessment of BMI and metabolic profile should be routine, with dietary counseling and CBT where appropriate. Among pharmacological interventions, adjunctive metformin has the best data, followed by topiramate.

Polypharmacy in Schizophrenia

REVIEW OF: Tiihonen J, Taipale H, Mehtälä J, et al. Association of antipsychotic polypharmacy vs monotherapy with psychiatric rehospitalization among adults with schizophrenia. *JAMA Psychiatry*. 2019 May 1;76(5):499–507.

Stroup TS, Gerhard T, Crystal S, et al. Comparative effectiveness of adjunctive psychotropic medications in patients with schizophrenia. *JAMA Psychiatry*. 2019 May 1;76(5):508–515.

ANTIPSYCHOTIC POLYPHARMACY IS discouraged in guidelines but common in practice. Up to 30% of patients with schizophrenia are prescribed multiple antipsychotics, and combinations of antipsychotics with other drug classes are even more common. Research on these practices, though, is sparse. Two recent studies, both large retrospective non-randomized controlled trials, attempted to clarify whether polypharmacy brings greater benefits in schizophrenia, or just greater risks.

STUDY ONE: Retrospective cohort study

The first study collected data from a population-wide registry in Finland on 62,250 patients with schizophrenia who were hospitalized and followed between 1996 and 2015 (median age 46; male to female ratio equal).

Hazard ratios (HR) were calculated by comparing patients on one, multiple, or no antipsychotics. Within-individual analysis was used to eliminate selection bias (ie, patients were their own controls). Of the total cohort, 67% used antipsychotic polypharmacy at some point. To exclude switches between antipsychotics, data from the first 90 days of multiple antipsychotic use were censored. The primary outcome was psychiatric rehospitalization, and secondary outcomes were mortality and medical hospitalization.

RESULTS

The risk of psychiatric rehospitalization was 13% lower with polypharmacy than monotherapy (HR 0.87; CI 0.85–0.88). That risk was lowest with the combination of clozapine and aripiprazole: 58% lower than no antipsychotic use (HR 0.42; CI 0.39–0.46) and 14% lower than clozapine alone (HR 0.86; CI 0.79–0.94). Among the top 10 treatments with the lowest risk of rehospitalization, only one was monotherapy: clozapine. Remarkably, polypharmacy was also associated with a lower risk of hospitalization due to medical illness and mortality.

STUDY TWO: Retrospective cohort study

The second study evaluated the effects of adding different drug classes to standard treatment in schizophrenia. Using a Medicaid registry, 81,921 patients with schizophrenia on antipsychotic therapy were followed for 1 year after starting an additional psychotropic (mean age 41; 54% male). Patients who were already on multiple psychiatric medications or who filled their antipsychotic inconsistently were excluded from the sample (n = 241 and 579).

HRs were calculated by comparing patients based on whether they were prescribed antidepressants, benzodiazepines, or mood stabilizers vs additional antipsychotics. Patients in each of the treatment groups were demographically similar. Those who did not start a new psychotropic were not included in the comparisons, as it was thought they represented a group with fewer comorbidities and better prognosis. Dropouts were handled by analyzing data on an intent-to-treat basis. The primary outcome was psychiatric hospitalization, and secondary outcomes included medical hospitalization and mortality.

RESULTS

The risk of psychiatric hospitalization was 16% lower for patients who started an antidepressant (HR 0.84; CI 0.80–0.88). Patients started on benzodiazepines had a higher risk of psychiatric hospitalization (HR 1.08; CI 1.02–1.15), while those started on mood stabilizers had an equal risk (HR 0.98; CI 0.94–1.03). Antidepressants were associated with a lower risk of medical hospitalization (HR 0.87; CI 0.79–0.96), whereas no difference was found for benzodiazepines or mood stabilizers. Mood stabilizers were the only group associated with a statistically higher risk of mortality (HR 1.31; CI 1.04–1.66), and this risk was highest with gabapentin.

THE CARLAT TAKE

Both studies had similar weaknesses. With the lack of randomization, various confounding variables could have been overlooked. Factors not examined include reasons for changing medications, frequency of patient-provider contact, use of psychosocial interventions, and extent of medication adherence. Functioning and symptom severity were also not examined. On the other hand, patients prescribed multiple psychotropics are likely to have lower functioning and greater disease severity, so the fact these patients had favorable outcomes is impressive.

PRACTICE IMPLICATIONS

Polypharmacy is often looked down on, but these results suggest it may be a viable strategy in schizophrenia. In combining antipsychotics, the best outcome was with clozapine and aripiprazole. This suggests prescribing antipsychotics with different receptor profiles may be a useful tactic. In terms of combining antipsychotics with other psychotropics, the results are even less definitive and more likely skewed. That limitation aside, antidepressants appear to have the greatest benefit and least risk. In contrast, mood stabilizers and benzodiazepines should be used with more caution.

An Answer for Psychotic Depression

REVIEW OF: **Flint AJ, Meyers BS, Rothschild AJ, et al. Effect of continuing olanzapine vs placebo on relapse among patients with psychotic depression in remission: The STOP-PD II randomized clinical trial.** *JAMA.* **2019 Aug 20;322(7):622–631.**

STUDY TYPE: **Randomized, double-blind, placebo-controlled trial**

PSYCHOTIC FEATURES IN depression indicate a more severe form of the disease, with a higher risk of hospitalization and double the rate of disability compared with non-psychotic depression. A combination of an antipsychotic and an antidepressant is the mainstay of treatment, but how long to continue the antipsychotic is an unanswered question.

This study enrolled patients 18–85 years of age with severe major depression and at least 1 delusion; hallucinations were optional. Dementia and unstable medical illness were part of the exclusion criteria, so the patients may not have been as ill as some whom we see in clinical practice. Average age was 55 years.

Researchers first treated 269 patients with open-label olanzapine and sertraline. Next, 162 patients who achieved remission or near-remission entered an open-label 8-week stabilization phase. Of the 147 who remained well after the stabilization, 126 were randomized to continue olanzapine or have the antipsychotic replaced with a placebo for 36 weeks. The design was double-blind, and the antipsychotic taper took place over 4 weeks. All patients remained on sertraline throughout the trial.

RESULTS

The primary outcome was risk of relapse, which included relapses into depression or psychosis as well as psychiatric hospitalization or suicidality. 55% of sertraline-placebo patients relapsed, compared to 20% of sertraline-olanzapine patients. The number needed to treat (NNT) to keep patients well with continued antipsychotic therapy was 2.8, which is a relatively low (favorable) value for depression treatment in general.

Weight gain was the main side effect of continued olanzapine. The placebo group lost weight while the olanzapine group continued to gain, with a difference of 9 pounds between them at the end of the study. Falls were also greater in the olanzapine-continuation group (31% vs 18%).

THE CARLAT TAKE

The majority of the relapses (79%) occurred within the first 20 weeks of the 36-week randomization phase. In a letter to the editor, Klaus Munkholm and colleagues argued that these relapses may have been a withdrawal phenomenon. The authors of the study countered that their criteria for relapse shared little in common with known symptoms of antipsychotic withdrawal.

PRACTICE IMPLICATIONS

When a patient recovers from psychotic depression on an antidepressant and antipsychotic, we should continue both medications for at least 2 months as long as the medication is reasonably tolerable. After 6 months of remission (28 weeks), we might consider a slow taper of the antipsychotic, weighing the severity of the episode, side effects, and the patient's preferences.

ANXIETY DISORDERS

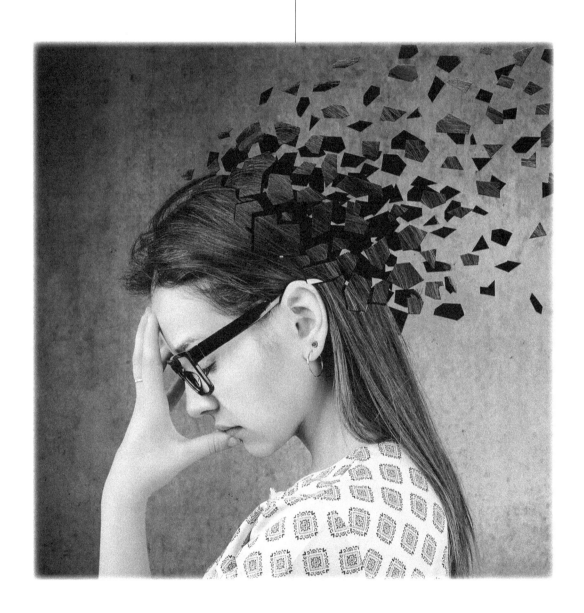

Pharmacology for GAD: Complex Choices

REVIEW OF: **Slee A, Nazareth I, Bondaronek P, et al. Pharmacological treatments for generalised anxiety disorder: A systematic review and network meta-analysis. *Lancet*. 2019 Feb 23;393(10173):768–777.**

STUDY TYPE: **Network meta-analysis**

WITH OVER TWO dozen choices, how do we pick a medication for generalized anxiety disorder (GAD)? The authors of this network meta-analysis sought to answer this question.

Network meta-analysis allows researchers to gauge treatments that haven't been directly compared in head-to-head studies. If drug A works better than drug B and B works better than C, then the network meta-analysis concludes that A is likely to work better than C, even though A and C have never been directly compared.

The investigators selected 89 trials of 25 drugs studied in over 25,000 patients. The primary outcome was change in the Hamilton Rating Scale for Anxiety (HAM-A). Trial length varied from 4 to 26 weeks.

RESULTS

Surprisingly, quetiapine XR was the most efficacious among the medications with large sample sizes. However, its benefit was modest, with a reduction of 3.6 points on the HAM-A compared to placebo (150–300 mg per night, as monotherapy). Quetiapine XR was poorly tolerated with a high discontinuation rate (odds ratio 1.44). The following drugs were well tolerated and are listed in order of efficacy: duloxetine, pregabalin, venlafaxine XR, and escitalopram.

The four benzodiazepines were studied as a class, not as individual drugs. Patients quit benzodiazepines much more often than placebo (odds ratio 1.43), although the reasons for discontinuation were not explored.

Studies were excluded if the patients had psychiatric comorbidities other than depression, which means the subjects might have been significantly less ill than the patients we see in routine practice. One-third of the trials were not placebo controlled, and a fairly large number of them had limited quality. However, a sensitivity analysis concluded that these deficiencies did not significantly distort the results.

THE CARLAT TAKE

Although the meta-analysis did not analyze the data according to the quality of the studies, dose, or duration of treatment, Carlat Publishing has analyzed these issues by drilling down on the appendix and the original studies. The studies of pregabalin were all of lower quality. The studies of duloxetine were of the highest quality, followed by escitalopram and venlafaxine XR. For duloxetine, venlafaxine, and escitalopram, high doses (eg, duloxetine 120 mg) were no more efficacious than medium doses (eg, duloxetine 60 mg). Of these three antidepressants, only venlafaxine XR was studied for more than 12 weeks, and those studies demonstrated greater efficacy than shorter studies, suggesting that its benefits may build over time.

PRACTICE IMPLICATIONS

In GAD, duloxetine stands out for its efficacy, safety, and the quality of its studies. This antidepressant has FDA approval in childhood GAD as well. It may take a few months to see the full effects of antidepressants in GAD, and medium doses are as likely to work as higher ones. Quetiapine XR is one of the more effective medications for GAD, but it has major safety and tolerability issues that caused the FDA to withhold its approval in 2009.

Is D-Cycloserine Useful for Panic Disorder Treatment Augmentation?

REVIEW OF: Hofmeijer-Sevink MK, Duits P, Rijkeboer MM, et al. No effects of D-cycloserine enhancement in exposure with response prevention therapy in panic disorder with agoraphobia: A double-blind, randomized controlled trial. *J Clin Psychopharmacol.* 2017 Oct;37(5):531–539.

STUDY TYPE: Randomized, double-blind, placebo-controlled trial

THE MAINSTAY OF current treatment for panic disorder involves SSRIs and psychotherapy, specifically either cognitive behavioral therapy (CBT) or exposure with response prevention (ERP) therapy. D-cycloserine (DCS) is a partial N-methyl-D-aspartate (NMDA) receptor agonist that may enhance extinction learning—the gradual decrease in the panic response during ERP. Several studies have evaluated whether adding DCS to ERP therapy might enhance the effectiveness of the therapy, but there have been mixed results.

Conducted at outpatient clinics at three mental health care institutions in the Netherlands, this study evaluated the effectiveness of adding DCS to panic disorder treatment. Fifty-seven patients with panic disorder and agoraphobia were randomized to one of three treatment arms: DCS before the ERP session, DCS after the ERP session, or placebo.

DCS or placebo was administered orally in a single 125 mg fixed dose, either at the beginning or the end of treatment, depending on the condition. All study participants underwent 12 weekly, 90-minute individual ERP sessions. The primary outcome was the mean score on the "alone" subscale of the Mobility Inventory (MI), which is a self-report tool used to measure agoraphobic avoidance behavior in various situations. Measurements were taken at baseline and during sessions 4, 8, and 12, and then at 3- and 6-month follow-up.

RESULTS

There was no difference in the primary outcome between those who received DCS (either pre- or post-ERP session) and placebo. However, within the two DCS treatment groups, the DCS post-ERP group showed a significant improvement in the primary outcome (p = 0.009; effect size = 0.6) measured at 3-month follow-up compared to the DCS pre-ERP group.

THE CARLAT TAKE

DCS augmentation of psychotherapy for anxiety disorders sounds plausible in theory, but many studies, including this one, don't show a significant difference when comparing DCS to placebo. However, the authors mention that this study had many limitations. First, the study may have been too small to show an effect—the researchers' power calculations called for 20 subjects per treatment arm, but only 19 were randomized to each arm. Second, the dosing of

125 mg of DCS may have been too high. This may sound illogical, but the way DCS is thought to work is by activating the NMDA receptor. At higher doses, though, DCS has partial NMDA receptor antagonist effects, which reduces its effect on extinction learning. Also, with higher doses and more administrations, patients are more likely to develop tolerance to DCS.

PRACTICE IMPLICATIONS

It's interesting that this study showed a small signal that DCS might be effective post-ERP treatment, but we'll need larger studies with more robust results before recommending that you start using DCS in your practice.

Prescribing Patterns for Children With Anxiety Disorders

REVIEW OF: **Bushnell GA, Compton SN, Dusetzina SB, et al. Treating pediatric anxiety: Initial use of SSRIs and other antianxiety prescription medications.** *J Clin Psychiatry*. 2018 Jan/Feb;79(1):16m11415.

STUDY TYPE: **Retrospective cohort study**

ANXIETY DISORDERS ARE some of the most common conditions we encounter in children and adolescents, and clinicians employ a variety of medications to treat them. This study examined prescribing patterns for the initial treatment of pediatric anxiety.

Researchers analyzed a large commercial claims database for information on patients ages 3–17 years who were diagnosed with an ICD-9 anxiety disorder (including OCD and PTSD) and started on an antianxiety medication between 2004 and 2014.

Overall, a majority of the 84,500 medicated patients were older teenagers, with 58% being 14–17, and 58% were female. Half of the patients (50%) were diagnosed with unspecified anxiety disorder. More than half received both a diagnosis and a prescription on the same day (57%). While 41% of patients had attended a psychotherapy session within the 30 days prior to medication initiation, it is unclear if the rest had seen a therapist in the past or were referred to one while being started on medications.

RESULTS

Unsurprisingly, most children were started on an SSRI (70%), while some received benzodiazepines (11%), hydroxyzine, guanfacine/clonidine, an atypical antipsychotic, or an antidepressant/antianxiety medication combination (3%–5% each). Children with OCD and selective mutism were more likely to be given SSRIs (83% and 82% respectively) as compared to those with panic disorder (54% SSRI, 30% benzodiazepine) or PTSD (53% SSRI, 14% atypical antipsychotic). Almost a third of children with no other recent psychiatric comorbidity were prescribed a non-SSRI. When compared to psychiatrists, primary care providers were more likely to prescribe non-SSRIs to kids with panic disorder and social phobia.

In a promising trend, across the decade of the study period, teens ages 14–17 were more likely to be started on SSRIs (55% in 2004 vs 65% in 2014) and less likely to be started on benzodiazepines (20% in 2004 vs 10% in 2014). SSRIs were more likely to be refilled after the first prescription (81%) as well as continued for at least 6 months (55%) as compared to benzodiazepines (25% and 5%) or atypical antipsychotics (71% and 41%). Moreover, almost a quarter of those who were initiated on benzodiazepines or atypical antipsychotics eventually got a prescription for an SSRI within 3 months.

THE CARLAT TAKE

Frequency of prescribing does not imply best practice for everyone. While SSRIs are the most commonly prescribed medications with the lowest discontinuation rates in this study, antipsychotics came second, and both have potentially significant side effects in context of a paucity of evidence-based research independent of manufacturer-sponsored studies, the lack of FDA support notwithstanding. It is good to see reductions in benzodiazepine use, as they have few truly legitimate indications (surgery, catatonia) and their potential short- and long-term risks in children and adolescents almost always outweigh their immediate benefits. Although devoid of FDA approval, medications like propranolol, hydroxyzine, and guanfacine/clonidine have an important role to play in mitigating acute anxiety episodes, as well as anxiety stemming from trauma, while minimizing risk of long-term adverse effects like metabolic syndrome.

PRACTICE IMPLICATIONS

SSRIs play an important role in treatment of childhood anxiety disorders, but as AACAP guidelines note, psychotherapy should be the first-line treatment, with medications considered in cases of moderate to severe anxiety or a lack of response or access to psychotherapy. Unless children and youth are equipped with anxiety management techniques, family and/or school interventions that reduce any relevant stressors, and psychotherapy that deals with underlying anxiety-provoking memories and schemata, then cessation of pharmacotherapy—even if partially or fully effective—is more likely to lead to relapse.

How Effective Are Medications
for Pediatric Anxiety?

REVIEW OF: **Strawn JR, Mills JA, Sauley BA, Welge JA. The impact of antidepressant dose and class on treatment response in pediatric anxiety disorders: A meta-analysis.** *J Am Acad Child Adolesc Psychiatry.* **2018 Apr;57(4):235–244.e2.**

STUDY TYPE: **Meta-analysis of randomized placebo-controlled trials**

ANTIDEPRESSANTS ARE PART of the first-line treatment for severe childhood anxiety disorders when removal of stressors and psychotherapy are not enough, but are all antidepressants created equal in this situation?

A recent meta-analysis shows that antidepressants have a moderate effect size of 0.56 for treating anxiety disorders in children (Locher C et al, *JAMA Psychiatry* 2017;74(10):1011–1020), but do we have the data to further break that down? Another meta-analysis was recently performed that can further guide us in tailoring our medication choices for pediatric anxiety disorders.

In this meta-analysis, the authors pooled data from nine randomized placebo-controlled trials that compared either an SSRI or an SNRI to placebo for the treatment of social, generalized, and/or separation anxiety disorders. Total sample size was 1,805 children ages 5–17 years, with 53% male. All studies were done in outpatient clinics and had a mix of federal and industry funding sources. The follow-up periods varied from 8 to 16 weeks, with a median of 10 weeks. Four SSRIs (fluoxetine, fluvoxamine, paroxetine, and sertraline) and three SNRIs (atomoxetine, venlafaxine, and duloxetine) were used in the studies. The primary outcomes were the time it took to see improvement, how treatment response differed between SSRIs and SNRIs, and differences in low-dose vs high-dose SSRIs. Rating scales, most commonly the Pediatric Anxiety Rating Scale (PARS), were administered every 2 weeks.

RESULTS

Overall, children improved quickly compared to placebo, with a statistically significant difference in the rating scales by week 2 ($p = 0.005$) and a clinically significant difference seen by week 6 ($p = 0.001$). SSRIs outperformed SNRIs over the entire treatment course, with a statistically significant difference emerging by week 2 ($p = 0.021$), but both classes of medications resulted in significant improvement compared to placebo by week 2. For the high-dose vs low-dose SSRI comparison, high-dose was considered > 1.5 fluoxetine equivalents (> 49.5 mg) per day. High-dose SSRI treatment resulted in earlier improvement (week 2), while low-dose treatment resulted in later improvement (week 6). However, over time, there was no significant difference between high-dose and low-dose treatment ($p = 0.638$), but the variance was greater for the low-dose group ($p < 0.001$).

THE CARLAT TAKE

This meta-analysis found that, overall, SSRIs resulted in greater improvement in childhood anxiety disorders than SNRIs, and that high-dose SSRIs led to earlier improvement. The authors postulate that the differences may be due to an underdeveloped noradrenergic system in children compared to the serotonergic system, or due to anxiety disorders themselves being caused by more dysfunction in the serotonergic system.

PRACTICE IMPLICATIONS

When making medication decisions, the more information we have, the better. This study confirms that both SSRIs and SNRIs are effective in treating pediatric anxiety disorders. And, all other things being equal, SSRIs may give better results. Unless you have a reason to avoid SSRIs, using them as the first-line medication choice makes sense. High-dose SSRIs may give faster results but may come at a cost of increased side effects. Always be on the lookout for activation (which is generally more common with SSRIs than SNRIs) and other side effects.

ADHD

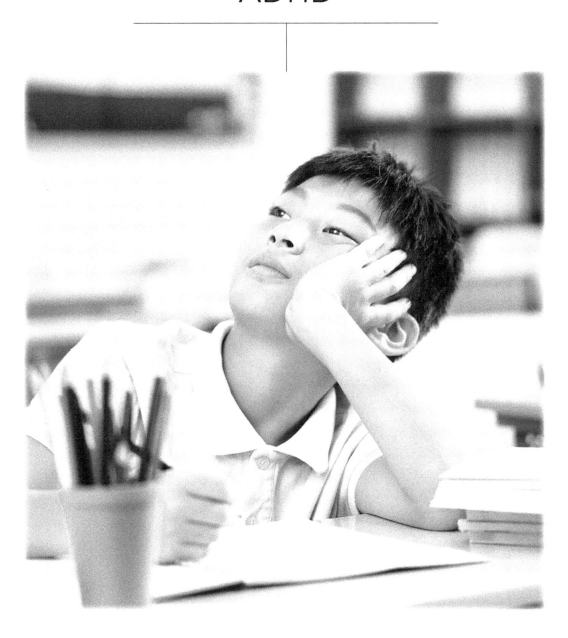

Risk of Psychosis With Stimulants in ADHD Patients

REVIEW OF: Moran LV, Ongur D, Hsu J, et al. Psychosis with methylphenidate or amphetamine in patients with ADHD. *N Engl J Med*. 2019 Mar 21;380(12):1128–1138.

STUDY TYPE: Retrospective cohort study

In 2007, the FDA required stimulant manufacturers to warn of possible psychosis with stimulants. But what is the real incidence of stimulant-induced psychosis? This study set out to discern if there is a difference between methylphenidate and amphetamine classes of medications in causing this potential adverse effect.

Drawing from two large commercial insurance databases, researchers looked at over 333,000 patients with ADHD ages 13–25 years who were prescribed a stimulant between 2004 and 2015, matching 110,923 methylphenidate users with an equal number of amphetamine users. The authors excluded patients with confounding variables (eg, glucocorticoid prescription) and adjusted for unmeasured confounders (eg, cannabis use). They defined "stimulant-induced psychosis" as a new psychotic illness within the follow-up period (median 4–5 months) along with a prescription for an antipsychotic within 60 days of that diagnosis.

RESULTS

Over the years 2005 to 2014, prescription of amphetamine salts increased 3.8 times, while that of methylphenidates increased only 1.6 times. It was notable that internists and family practice doctors tended to use amphetamines most often, prescribing amphetamines in 72.5% of stimulant prescriptions, with psychiatrists at 62.7% and pediatricians 51.6%.

The overall risk of psychosis was 1 in 660, with onset of psychotic symptoms occurring after a median 128 days. The risk in the amphetamine group was double compared to the methylphenidate group (237 episodes or 0.21% vs 106 episodes or 0.10%).

Amphetamine-related psychosis occurred more in younger children and those treated by non-psychiatrists (about 80% of patients). In the hands of internists and family practice doctors, the hazard ratio was 1.78, for pediatricians it was 1.7, and for psychiatrists it was 1.38.

THE CARLAT TAKE

Amphetamines, such as Adderall and Vyvanse, are more likely to lead to psychosis than methylphenidate, though the actual prevalence is quite low. Those children and young adults who were treated by psychiatrists had a lower rate of stimulant-induced psychosis.

PRACTICE IMPLICATIONS

We recommend extra caution in the use of stimulants (especially amphetamines) in those with other risk factors for psychosis (eg, family history of psychosis, cognitive or behavioral signs of prodromal psychosis, or concurrent cannabis use). In the broader picture, methylphenidate is usually better tolerated in any case and probably a better first-line medication.

How Helpful Is Computerized Testing for ADHD?

REVIEW OF: Hollis C, Hall CL, Guo B, et al. The impact of a computerised test of attention and activity (QbTest) on diagnostic decision-making in children and young people with suspected attention deficit hyperactivity disorder: Single-blind randomised controlled trial. *J Child Psychol Psychiatry*. 2018 Dec;59(12):1298–1308.

STUDY TYPE: Randomized, single-blind, active-controlled trial

WITH BUSY CLINIC schedules and the ever-burgeoning load of documentation, computerized diagnostic aids are in more demand than ever. For ADHD, the gold standard is still a clinical assessment with information from parents and teachers, but those reports are difficult to obtain and time-consuming to go through. In these situations, computerized testing may help boost clinical decision-making.

One common testing procedure is continuous performance testing (CPT), which involves a subject's ability to quickly respond to a given stimulus while not responding to distracting stimuli. QbTest is a specific testing method that combines computerized CPT and an infrared camera measuring how much the patient moves around during the 20-minute test. In 2014, the FDA cleared QbTest as a tool to supplement a clinical assessment for ADHD, meaning that it reached the diagnostic sensitivity and specificity thresholds required by the FDA. However, like all such tests, it is not meant to be a standalone diagnostic test. This study attempted to see how useful QbTest is for clinicians.

The randomized controlled trial analyzed data from 250 youth ages 6–17 years referred for an ADHD assessment. Funding came from the National Institute for Health Research in the UK, but equipment and training were provided directly from Qbtech Ltd (the makers of QbTest). The device's website (www.qbtech.com/qbtest) has descriptions of the testing equipment: an infrared camera, a reflector that fits on the patient's forehead, and the computer software. The sample, drawn from UK outpatient clinics, was nearly 80% male and 90% white. All participants took the QbTest at the beginning of the study period, then were divided into two groups. The QbOpen group had the results revealed to the clinician immediately, while the QbBlind group withheld the results. The primary outcome was the number of appointments it took to rule in or out an ADHD diagnosis, with secondary outcomes including appointment duration and clinician's confidence in the diagnosis.

RESULTS

At the end of 6 months, the youth in the QbOpen group were 44% more likely (hazard ratio = 1.44; p = 0.029) to have reached a diagnostic decision than those in the QbBlind group. However, over 30% of the entire sample had still not reached a diagnostic decision at 6 months. Interestingly, ADHD was excluded at double the rate when clinicians had access to the QbTest report (p = 0.049), and they were more confident in their decision overall (p = 0.022). The appointment duration for the QbOpen group was reduced by about 15% (p = 0.001). The authors also did a cost analysis concluding that QbTest was largely cost-neutral to the health care system.

THE CARLAT TAKE

As clinicians, we need to maintain diagnostic pre-eminence over supplemental tests for ADHD. While QbTest may increase the expediency of diagnosis and boost diagnostic confidence for clinicians, we need to be careful that it is neither masking other reasons for symptoms nor ruling them out when, for instance, the child being tested is inattentive but not overactive. It would also be interesting to see more comparison studies with more established measures such as the TOVA, GDS, IVA, or Connors CPT.

PRACTICE IMPLICATIONS

Computerized testing does not replace clinical assessments and collateral information from parents and teachers. While QbTest can provide some interesting information and more data points on which to base a diagnosis, it won't be putting anyone out of business.

Would Treating Kids With ADHD Help Their Mothers?

REVIEW OF: Gokcen C, Coskun S, Kutuk MO. Comparison of depression and burnout levels of mothers of children with attention-deficit hyperactivity disorder before and after treatment. *J Child Adolesc Psychopharmacol.* 2018 Jun;28(5):350–353.

STUDY TYPE: Prospective cohort study

PARENTING A CHILD with ADHD can be challenging. Parents often report feeling stressed, burned out, or depressed while caring for their children with ADHD. When ADHD medications lead to significant improvements in a child's behavior, can that alleviate symptoms in parents? A recently published study tried to examine that.

Investigators enrolled 40 children ages 4–10 years with ADHD at an outpatient clinic in Turkey. Twenty-one children completed the 8-week study and were prescribed methylphenidate (15), atomoxetine (3), or, surprisingly, risperidone (3). Researchers assessed the kids with a parent rating scale based on the DSM-IV criteria for ADHD, oppositional defiant disorder (ODD), and conduct disorder (CD) (Turgay-DSM-IV-S). They simultaneously assessed the kids' mothers for depression and burnout symptoms using Beck's Depression Inventory and the Maslach Burnout Inventory.

RESULTS

At the follow-up visit, the researchers found that children showed improvement in their scores of inattention (14.8±6.9 vs 11±8), hyperactivity (18±6.5 vs 10.5±8), ODD (11.6±6.4 vs 7.6±6.3), and CD (4.9±6.2 vs 2±3.7) symptoms. Moreover, their mothers also showed improvement in depression (14.5±7.7 vs 10.4±6.5) and burnout (18.3±10.6 vs 13±9.5). Interestingly, the improvement in mothers' burnout symptoms correlated with kids' ODD and CD symptoms (r = 0.5 and p = 0.02 for both), and improvement in mothers' depression symptoms correlated with CD symptoms in kids (r = 0.47; p = 0.03). Changes in mothers' symptoms did not correlate with the changes in children's inattention and hyperactivity symptoms.

THE CARLAT TAKE

This study suggests that improvement in ODD and CD symptoms in children with ADHD is associated with a decrease in burnout and depression symptoms in mothers. However, the findings of this study are difficult to generalize due to small sample size (40), high dropout rate (47.5%), lack of a control group, and an unclear separation between the pre-treatment and post-treatment scores. Furthermore, the authors did not disclose the rationale or dosage for the medications selected; they also did not disclose the psychiatric treatment status of the mothers.

PRACTICE IMPLICATIONS

When evaluating a child for ADHD symptoms, comorbid disorders like ODD and CD must be assessed and addressed appropriately. Whether or not this study proves causation, it makes sense that improvement in ODD and CD domains in children with ADHD can lead to all-around healthier families and communities.

Amphetamine Extended-Release Oral Suspension for ADHD

REVIEW OF: Childress AC, Wigal SB, Brams MN, et al. Efficacy and safety of amphetamine extended-release oral suspension in children with attention-deficit/hyperactivity disorder. *J Child Adolesc Psychopharmacol.* 2018 Jun;28(5):306–313.

STUDY TYPE: Randomized, double-blind, placebo-controlled trial

IN 2015, THE FDA approved Dyanavel XR (amphetamine extended-release oral suspension), which was the first long-acting liquid version of amphetamine on the market. To provide some context, Quillivant XR, a long-acting liquid methylphenidate formulation, was approved in 2012 and appears to be fairly popular for kids who can't or won't swallow pills. Seeing a market opportunity, Tris Pharmaceuticals developed Dyanavel XR and funded a placebo-controlled trial that was successful enough to gain FDA approval. Recently, this study was published, and some readers might be curious to look at the quality of the data.

The study took place at five investigational sites in the US. A total of 108 boys and girls with ADHD (ages 6–12) were initially enrolled in a 5-week open-label phase in which all patients were given Dyanavel XR, starting at 2.5–5 mg and titrated up to a target dose of 10–20 mg/day. Nine children dropped out of this first phase, and 99 continued on to the placebo-controlled phase of the study. Participants were randomly assigned to either Dyanavel XR (51 patients, mean dose 17.3 mg) or placebo (48 patients). After 1 week on the medication, the children's ADHD symptoms were evaluated with a teacher-rated instrument called the SKAMP (for the Swanson, Kotkin, Agler, M-Flynn, and Pelham Rating Scale).

RESULTS

The primary outcome variable was improvement in SKAMP scores from pre-dose to post-dose of medication. Dyanavel XR was more effective than placebo beginning 1 hour after the dose and continuing for 13 hours. The effect size was a very robust 1.8, in line with effect sizes reported in similar trials of other long-acting stimulants. In terms of side effects, patients on Dyanavel XR reported decreased appetite (26%), insomnia (13%), and affect lability (9%), with no substantial differences in blood pressure or pulse between the treatment and control group.

THE CARLAT TAKE

Not too surprisingly, Dyanavel XR is an effective stimulant treatment for ADHD. This study was not huge but was well designed, and the results were judged to be robust enough to merit FDA approval.

PRACTICE IMPLICATIONS

Dyanavel XR is another arrow in our ever-expanding quiver of stimulant options, and this liquid formulation will likely be just as popular as methylphenidate's liquid XR: Quillivant, first approved in 2012 for ADHD treatment. Being a brand-name option, its cost is high. For families that want cheaper liquid stimulants, go with either generic ProCentra (short-acting dextroamphetamine) or Methylin oral solution (short-acting methylphenidate).

Amphetamines Stand Out in ADHD

REVIEW OF: **Cortese S, Adamo N, Del Giovane C, et al. Comparative efficacy and tolerability of medications for attention-deficit hyperactivity disorder in children, adolescents, and adults: A systematic review and network meta-analysis.** *Lancet Psychiatry.* **2018 Sep;5(9):727–738.**

STUDY TYPE: **Meta-analysis of randomized controlled trials**

WITH SO MANY medications available to treat ADHD, wouldn't it be nice to know if some are better than others? In this comprehensive meta-analysis, researchers sought to compare the relative efficacy and tolerability of both stimulant (methylphenidate and amphetamines) and non-stimulant (atomoxetine, bupropion, modafinil, clonidine, and guanfacine) medications for ADHD in children and adults.

The investigators combed through published and unpublished databases and located 82 double-blind, randomized controlled trials in children and adolescents, and 52 such trials in adults. Together, they included over 10,000 children and adolescents, and over 8,000 adults. The primary outcome was change in clinician-rated ADHD symptoms, while teacher ratings were also evaluated for children. "Tolerability" was defined as the percentage who dropped out because of side effects, while the broader term "acceptability" referred to those who dropped out for any reason. Outcomes were evaluated through 12 weeks of treatment.

RESULTS

In children and adolescents, all medications were superior to placebo. Amphetamines emerged as the most effective ADHD medication, superior to modafinil, guanfacine, atomoxetine, and methylphenidate. Methylphenidate was superior to atomoxetine. Based on teacher ratings, only methylphenidate and modafinil separated from placebo (none of the amphetamine trials included teacher ratings). With respect to tolerability, amphetamines and guanfacine both displayed significantly more adverse effects than placebo; amphetamines also significantly increased diastolic blood pressure. Methylphenidate was better tolerated than the amphetamines, and it was the only medication with better acceptability than placebo.

In adults, amphetamines emerged not only as the most efficacious agents but also the only ones with better acceptability than placebo. Methylphenidate, atomoxetine, and bupropion all had similar effect sizes. Modafinil was ineffective in adults, despite having positive results in children. At the time of this analysis, there were no trials of the alpha-2A agonists (clonidine ER and guanfacine ER) in adults, but a more recent randomized placebo-controlled trial did find favorable results for guanfacine ER in 108 adult patients with ADHD (Iwanami A et al, *J Clin Psychiatry* 2020;81(3):19m12979).

Tolerability was similar among the agents. In contrast to their effects on children, amphetamines did not increase diastolic blood pressure in adults. Overall, ADHD medications were less efficacious and less well tolerated in adults than in children and adolescents.

THE CARLAT TAKE

This meta-analysis seems to give us more reason to prescribe amphetamines, but there was a dearth of head-to-head trials, so these comparisons could only be made indirectly. The dropout rate was used as a proxy for acceptability, and this is a rough estimate. Finally, while the large sample sizes instill greater confidence in the results, they also risk finding significant differences that may not necessarily be clinically meaningful.

PRACTICE IMPLICATIONS

One medication rarely stands out in its class, but the amphetamines clearly emerged as the most effective option in both children and adults. That does not mean they should always be first choice, though. Methylphenidate was a more tolerable option in children, and there will always be patients who respond better to the methylphenidate varieties. Non-stimulant options take longer to work, but they performed fairly well in this meta-analysis, sometimes rivaling methylphenidate's benefits. The only failure was modafinil, which worked in children but not adults.

Can Stimulants Prevent Crime?

REVIEW OF: **Mohr-Jensen C, Bisgaard CM, Boldsen SK, Steinhausen HC. Attention-deficit/hyperactivity disorder in childhood and adolescence and the risk of crime in young adulthood in a Danish nationwide study. *J Am Acad Child Adolesc Psychiatry*. 2019 Apr;58(4):443–452.**

STUDY TYPE: **Retrospective case-control series**

ADHD HAS LONG been linked to antisocial behavior leading to arrests and incarcerations. Children and young adults with ADHD are more likely to be charged with anything from traffic violations to violent crimes. However, these associations do not prove causality. Is the ADHD causing these antisocial behaviors, or are there other psychosocial factors that would explain the findings? And if ADHD is indeed an independent risk factor for criminal behavior, can that risk be decreased through stimulant medication?

These big questions require population-based studies. Researchers evaluated data from Danish national medical and prescription registries and matched 4,231 children diagnosed with ADHD from 1995 to 2005, with controls based on sex and age. Follow-up data from an average of 22 years were obtained regarding arrests, incarcerations, substance abuse, time on stimulant medications, and other psychosocial factors. Nearly all (98%) of stimulant prescriptions were for methylphenidate, and most of the children (85%) were male.

RESULTS

After controlling for confounders such as psychiatric comorbidity, socioeconomic status, parental psychopathology, and other psychosocial factors, males with ADHD were 60% more likely (hazard ratio [HR] = 1.6) to be convicted of a crime and 70% more likely (HR = 1.7) to be incarcerated. For females, the effect was even more profound—they were 120% more likely (HR = 2.2) to be convicted and 190% more likely (HR = 2.9) to be incarcerated. However, when looking at times of active treatment with stimulant medication, the risk of conviction dropped significantly by 40% (HR = 0.6) for both males and females compared to time periods off medication. Incarceration risk also dropped by 40% (HR = 0.6) for males but did not drop significantly for females.

THE CARLAT TAKE

This study takes a mile-high view of a given population, looking for large trends over time. While population-based studies do not apply to every individual patient, knowing that appropriate treatment of ADHD may prevent criminal behavior is very encouraging.

PRACTICE IMPLICATIONS

The data for more severe consequences of ADHD in females are particularly interesting, though they may stem from underrecognized mild ADHD in girls. For all cases, early recognition of the complex needs (related to poverty, trauma, etc.) of children with ADHD and supporting psychosocial treatment with medication can change lives.

Methylphenidate Max Dosing

REVIEW OF: Ching C, Eslick GD, Poulton AS. Evaluation of methylphenidate safety and maximum-dose titration rationale in attention-deficit/hyperactivity disorder: A meta-analysis. *JAMA Pediatr.* 2019 Jul 1;173(7):630–639.

STUDY TYPE: Meta-analysis of randomized controlled trials

METHYLPHENIDATE WAS ONE of the first stimulants prescribed for the treatment of ADHD in children, adolescents, and adults. Its efficacy is clear, and its availability in immediate release, sustained release, osmotic-release oral system (OROS, brand name Concerta), and transdermal patch keeps it a popular choice. The typical dosing strategy in children and adolescents is to start low and go slow, but if symptoms remain and side effects are tolerable, at what dose should we stop titrating?

The standard FDA dosing information recommends a maximum dose of 60 mg per day in children and adolescents ages 6–17 for both immediate-release and sustained-release methylphenidate. For the OROS formulation, the dose is capped at 54 mg per day for children ages 6–12 and 72 mg per day in adolescents ages 13–17. These guidelines are backed by a few randomized controlled trials, and various organizations have slightly different maximum dose guidelines, but does the rest of the literature support these limits?

RESULTS

This meta-analysis reviewed data from 11 randomized controlled trials (1,304 participants) and 38 cohort studies (5,524 participants) examining methylphenidate dosing strategies. Some studies cited guidelines or previous studies for their maximum doses, but several of the studies capped themselves at a lower maximum dose than the source they were citing recommended. Most studies listed maximum doses far lower than the common guidelines. Only one cohort study went higher—90 mg per day of OROS for ages 6–13. Overall adverse effects were common at a rate of 66% in the cohort studies. The most common side effects were decreased appetite (33%), insomnia (15%), and headaches (14%). Serious adverse events were exceedingly rare, with transient psychosis reported in just 5 cohort study participants and hypertension in 7.

THE CARLAT TAKE

There is ample evidence of efficacy for many patients at dosages lower than the suggested maximums, yet evidence for a true maximum dose for methylphenidate is lacking. The variability in each patient's pharmacokinetics argues for an individualized dosing scheme that may lead to a lower or higher dose as needed (Childress AC et al, *Expert Opin Drug Metab Toxicol* 2019;15(11):937–974).

PRACTICE IMPLICATIONS

If a patient's ADHD symptoms remain on a given dose, and a review of the differential diagnosis yields no other intercurrent conditions, we do not have evidence that would preclude continued careful upward titration of stimulant medications while monitoring for side effects.

CHILD AND ADOLESCENT PSYCHIATRY

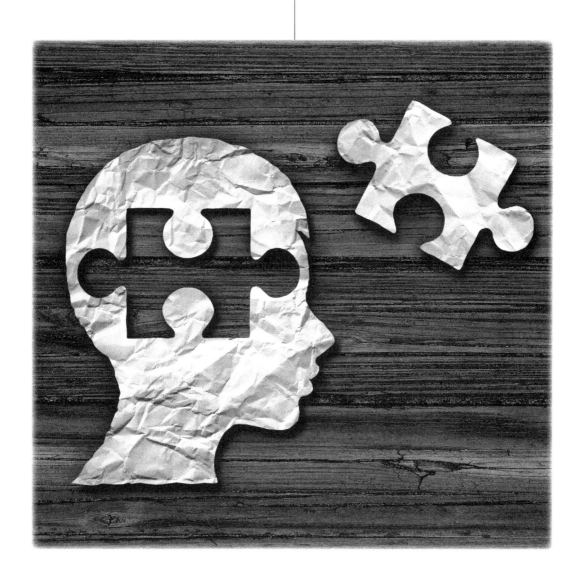

Melatonin for Insomnia in Patients With Autism

REVIEW OF: **Maras A, Schroder CM, Malow BA, et al. Long-term efficacy and safety of pediatric prolonged-release melatonin for insomnia in children with autism spectrum disorder. *J Child Adolesc Psychopharmacol.* 2018 Dec;28(10):699–710.**

STUDY TYPE: **Open-label extension of a randomized placebo-controlled trial**

TREATING SLEEP PROBLEMS in youth with autism spectrum disorder (ASD) is tricky at best. One promising treatment is pediatric prolonged-release melatonin (PedPRM) sold under the name Slenyto. In 2017, a randomized controlled trial (funded by the manufacturer) assigned 119 children with ASD and insomnia to either PedPRM (n = 58) or placebo (n = 61). PedPRM outperformed placebo: 68.9% of patients taking the medication had improved sleep outcomes vs only 39.3% of those assigned to placebo (p = 0.001).

Now a new article has been published to determine whether PedPRM maintains its effectiveness over the long term. A total of 95 patients entered this open-label phase, and 84% (n = 80) completed the phase. The average age of the patients was 9 years, and 75% were male. Youths previously randomized to placebo were switched to PedPRM and titrated to a maximum dose of 10 mg/day. Average dose was 8.3 mg for adolescents and 5.6 mg for younger children.

RESULTS

After 37 weeks, children originally randomized to and maintained on PedPRM showed sustained improvements: shorter sleep latency, greater length of sleep, fewer awakenings, and better sleep quality. In addition, those who previously received placebo showed improvement in sleep length and onset after switching to PedPRM. Caregivers' quality of life improved as well, with 49% of caregivers experiencing an improvement on the quality-of-life scale used in the study.

The most common side effect of PedPRM was daytime fatigue, which occurred in 18% of the patients. There were no serious adverse events attributed to the medication, including aggression.

THE CARLAT TAKE

This industry-funded study reports compelling results, which begs us to presume bias despite what appears to be sound methodology. It would be helpful to see a head-to-head study vs over-the-counter melatonin, which is cheaper albeit with more pill-to-pill variability. A more recent study from the same group in 2020 again reported efficacy of prolonged-release melatonin in children with ASD without significant impacts on growth and pubertal development (Malow BA et al, *J Am Acad Child Adolesc Psychiatry* 2020;S0890-8567(20)30034-4).

PRACTICE IMPLICATIONS

Despite the possible industry bias, PedPRM may be a viable treatment option for children with autism and insomnia. However, first-line treatment is still a comprehensive sleep hygiene approach including attention to sensory issues, daily exercise, and psychotherapy, all of which might be effective for insomnia in this population.

Rapid-Onset Gender Dysphoria in Adolescents and Young Adults

REVIEW OF: Littman L. Parent reports of adolescents and young adults perceived to show signs of a rapid onset of gender dysphoria. *PLoS One*. 2018 Aug 16;13(8):e0202330.

STUDY TYPE: Cross-sectional study

RAPID-ONSET GENDER DYSPHORIA (ROGD) is a newly coined but non-standardized characterization of gender dysphoria (GD). In this conceptualization, GD begins abruptly during or after puberty in adolescents or young adults (AYAs) with no prior symptoms of GD. Clusters of GD outbreaks have been noted by parents. These outbreaks have occurred in preexisting friend groups in which members became GD or identified as transgender. ROGD is often preceded by an immersion in social media.

Littman studied this phenomenon further. She placed a link to a 90-question survey, consisting of multiple-choice, Likert-type, and open-ended questions, on three websites where parents had reported ROGD. These websites were all notable in that they questioned the medicalization of gender-atypical youth. Data were collected anonymously via SurveyMonkey.

RESULTS

Overall, 256 parents completed questionnaires meeting study criteria. The sample of AYAs was predominantly white, academically gifted, and female sex at birth (82.8%) with a mean age of 16.4 years. Data collected included:

- Many AYAs (62.5%) were diagnosed with at least 1 mental health disorder prior to the onset of GD. Anxiety (63.4%) and depression (58.8%) were the most common. Nearly half of the group had engaged in self-harm.
- Several had experienced a family stressor (44.2%) or sex-/gender-related trauma (30%) prior to the onset of GD.
- 30% of AYAs were not willing to work on their mental health needs before seeking gender treatment.
- For parents who knew the content of their child's GD evaluation, alarmingly, 71.6% reported that the clinician did not explore issues of mental health, previous trauma, or alternative contributors to GD before continuing. 70.0% reported the clinician did not request any medical records.

THE CARLAT TAKE

It is encouraging that individuals who previously might have been underdiagnosed and undertreated are now gaining visibility. It can take tremendous courage to come out as transgender. Still, this study is controversial; *PLoS One* even engaged in a year-long second peer review period prior to this publication. These findings are important to take in context, including the potential for bias in the sampling of parent views, not teens, and specific websites that carry a cause, as well as the usual caveat that such data cannot be seen as causative per se. This study had quite a few responses that questioned the parent-only interviews and prompted a re-publication in 2019 emphasizing the observational nature of the study (Littman L, *PLoS One* 2019;14(3):e0214157). Littman states that the study had no comparison group and wasn't meant to test a hypothesis but to generate possible hypotheses regarding gender dysphoria in AYAs.

PRACTICE IMPLICATIONS

As clinicians, we need to identify trauma and psychopathology, and we need to manage those difficulties before addressing the AYA's decision regarding sex reassignment or gender transition. Online content and friend groups may influence susceptible AYAs to believe that other psychological distress should be understood as GD. Some AYAs are engaged in online interactions where they are coached in what to say to clinicians, perhaps misrepresenting symptoms, in order to obtain their desired treatment. As a result, it is vital to gather information from collateral informants, including parents, pediatricians, and therapists, and to consider the role of such things as peer interactions, media influences, abuse, family dynamics, and psychodynamic processes.

We would do well to encourage AYAs and parents to allow time for the process to unfold. It may then become clearer whether the symptoms are stable versus an expression of other clinical distress.

Effects of *13 Reasons Why* on Teens

REVIEW OF: Bridge JA, Greenhouse JB, Ruch D, et al. Association between the release of Netflix's *13 Reasons Why* and suicide rates in the United States: An interrupted time series analysis. *J Am Acad Child Adolesc Psychiatry.* 2020 Feb;59(2):236–243.

STUDY TYPE: Cross-sectional study

NETFLIX's *13 REASONS Why* (13RW) continues to generate controversy that it may do more harm than good amid the backdrop of an already increasing teen suicide rate. In previous research updates we reported an increased suicide rate in 10- to 19-year-old females during the 3 months following the show's 2017 premiere (Niederkrotenthaler T et al, *JAMA Psychiatry* 2019;76(9):933–940). Let's look at a second, similarly designed study.

Investigators examined CDC-collected suicide and homicide data before and after the show's release in April 2017. Data were assessed across 5 years (2013–2017) and these age groups: 10–17 years, 18–29 years, and 30–64 years.

RESULTS

Among the show's target audience (ages 10–17), suicide counts were 28.9% higher than expected in the first month following the series premiere. No excess suicide mortality was found in other age groups or in the control outcome, homicide counts. Overall, there were an additional 195 suicide deaths among 10- to 17-year-olds in the 9 months following the premiere. Suicides beyond expected rates were higher in boys than in girls. (Of note, season 1 depicts a male adolescent character making a serious suicide attempt by firearm.) Further, the authors used data showing suicide completion: Adolescent girls are 3 times more likely to attempt suicide than boys, but boys are 4 times more likely to complete suicide.

THE CARLAT TAKE

We now have two epidemiological studies that found associations between the release of *13RW* and increased youth suicides: the 2019 *JAMA Psychiatry* study finding a higher rate in girls, this study finding a higher rate in boys. Each study supports potential suicide contagion by media, at least for season 1, based on timing and age specificity. Netflix has since taken measures to try to reduce risk such as adding content warnings, removing the season 1 suicide scene, and publishing an online toolkit for clinicians, parents, youth, educators, and media professionals (www.13reasonswhytoolkit.org). The toolkit summarizes research outcomes from *13RW*, counsels that at-risk youth should not watch the series, and cautions against teen binge-watching. It also recommends that if teens watch the show, they should do so with a parent or trusted adult and engage in discussions around viewing risk and how to recognize and seek help for negative reactions, if they occur. This is crucial given the recent release of the series' fourth and final season.

PRACTICE IMPLICATIONS

Based on this growing research, it seems apparent that *13RW* may be particularly problematic for at-risk youths. As mental health providers, we need to be aware of this association and provide psychoeducation to youth and families. Our role includes urging parental engagement and advocating for treatment for at-risk youth, while admonishing the media to value life over profits. Mental health provider criticisms about the show's content and associated risk led to Netflix's aforementioned changes, demonstrating the impact of our collective voices. The situation warrants continued surveillance on suicide rates in association with viewing the series, particularly as a fourth season was released in June 2020.

Simvastatin as Adjunctive Therapy for Irritability in Autism

REVIEW OF: Moazen-Zadeh E, Shirzad F, Karkhaneh-Yousefi MA, et al. Simvastatin as an adjunctive therapy to risperidone in treatment of autism: A randomized, double-blind, placebo-controlled clinical trial. *J Child Adolesc Psychopharmacol.* **2018 Feb;28(1):82–89.**

STUDY TYPE: Randomized, double-blind, placebo-controlled trial

DISORDERS OF LIPID metabolism—specifically inefficient metabolism of lipids—have been implicated as part of the metabolic complexity in children with autism spectrum disorder. Research points to the neuroprotective effects of simvastatin over other statins, due to its greater ability to cross the blood-brain barrier. But does that neuroprotection translate to differences in behavior? This trial compared simvastatin to placebo as adjunctive treatment to risperidone for irritability in children meeting criteria for DSM-IV-TR autistic disorder (AD).

All participants scored ≥ 12 on the Aberrant Behavior Checklist-Community (ABC-C) irritability subscale, and therefore met criteria for treatment of irritability with medications. The ABC-C scale rates children on 58 items arranged in five behavioral abnormality subscales. In total, 66 children ages 4–12 years completed the trial and were randomized to receive risperidone and either simvastatin or placebo. Risperidone target dose was 1 mg/day if < 20 kg and 2 mg/day if ≥ 20 kg. Simvastatin was started concurrently with risperidone and was dosed at 20 mg/day for children < 10 years old and 40 mg/day if ≥ 10 years old. The ABC-C rating scale was assessed at baseline, week 5, and week 10.

RESULTS

The primary outcome was change in the ABC-C irritability subscale, which showed a significant difference in favor of the simvastatin arm at week 10 (−3.45; p = 0.001). Secondary outcomes were the other four subscales, for which there was a significant improvement in the simvastatin group over placebo only in the hyperactivity/noncompliance subscale (−4.27; p = 0.001).

The other subscales that represent the core deficits of AD (lethargy/social withdrawal, stereotypic behavior, and inappropriate speech) showed no significant differences. There was also no significant difference in any adverse events between the groups. The more common side effects across both groups were increased appetite (25.8%), myalgia (13.6%), nausea (12.1%), and headache (12.1%).

THE CARLAT TAKE

The results of this study are promising, but it is only the first of its kind to evaluate simvastatin treatment in this clinical setting. Anti-inflammatory treatments are showing promise in a wide range of psychiatric illnesses, but the core symptoms of autism remain difficult to treat with any type of therapy.

PRACTICE IMPLICATIONS

Since long-term benefits or adverse effects have not been established, it's too early to recommend using simvastatin as a treatment of autism. As in studies of anti-inflammatory interventions, behavioral symptoms may be improved, but the core symptoms of autism remain unchanged.

Azithromycin for Acute-Onset Obsessive-Compulsive Disorder in Children

REVIEW OF: Murphy TK, Brennan EM, Johnco C, et al. A double-blind randomized placebo-controlled pilot study of azithromycin in youth with acute-onset obsessive-compulsive disorder. *J Child Adolesc Psychopharmacol.* 2017 Sep;27(7):640–651.

STUDY TYPE: Randomized, double-blind, placebo-controlled trial

PEDIATRIC ACUTE-ONSET NEUROPSYCHIATRIC syndrome (PANS) and pediatric autoimmune neuropsychiatric syndrome associated with streptococcus (PANDAS) have been the subject of many debates in the field. From obsessions, compulsions, and tics, to personality changes and oppositional behavior, the symptoms of PANS are wide ranging. PANDAS is considered a subset of PANS that is temporally associated with a Group A streptococcal (GAS) infection.

Due to the link to an infectious cause, antibiotics are being assessed as a treatment for PANS. This study specifically evaluated the tolerability and efficacy of azithromycin in treating children with acute onset of OCD who met criteria for PANS.

Conducted with 31 children ages 4–14, the study compared treatment with azithromycin (10 mg/kg, up to 500 mg per day) to placebo for children with an acute onset of moderate or worse OCD symptoms and neuropsychiatric symptoms. The primary outcomes were changes in the Children's Yale-Brown Obsessive Compulsive Scale (CY-BOCS), and in the Clinical Global Impression—Severity (CGI-S) scale. Several secondary outcomes were measured, including other scales for tic severity, affective lability, and anxiety. Outcome measurements were taken at baseline and then weekly for 4 weeks over the study period.

RESULTS

The results of the trial were split. The azithromycin group had a significantly greater reduction in OCD severity as measured by the CGI-S ($p = 0.003$) at week 4, but there was no significant difference between the treatment and control groups in the CY-BOCS scores ($p = 0.203$). Interestingly, the children in the azithromycin group with greater tic severity at baseline showed the most improvement in the CGI-S. For the secondary outcome measures, the only significant effect was a reduction in the Clinical Global Impression—Improvement Mood subscale ($p = 0.006$) in the azithromycin group.

As for side effects, the azithromycin group had significantly more loose stools (53% of treatment group vs 7% of placebo group), and the placebo group reported more constipation (36% of placebo group vs 0% of treatment group). Electrocardiograms were monitored at baseline and at week 4, showing a significant increase in the QTc ($p = 0.007$) for children in the azithromycin group. Four participants in the azithromycin group had a borderline QTc of 440–460 at week 4 versus 1 participant in the placebo group.

THE CARLAT TAKE

This study, along with other past trials of antibiotics for PANS, gives us mixed results. The authors postulate that the CY-BOCS may not have been the best rating tool for the younger children in this trial, leading to the less robust results compared to the CGI-S outcome. Better response to antibiotic treatment was mediated by baseline tic severity, which will need further exploration.

PRACTICE IMPLICATIONS

This small study is best viewed as a pilot that may lead to larger trials in the future. If you consider using azithromycin for acute-onset OCD, weigh this against the potential for promoting antibiotic resistance and for severe potential side effects such as pseudomembranous colitis, and if you proceed with treatment, you may want to obtain baseline and follow-up electrocardiograms to watch for QTc changes.

Engage Those Infants: Maternal Interaction and Autism

REVIEW OF: Schwichtenberg AJ, Kellerman AM, Young GS, Miller M, Ozonoff S. Mothers of children with autism spectrum disorders: Play behaviors with infant siblings and social responsiveness. *Autism*. 2019 May;23(4):821–833.

STUDY TYPE: Prospective cohort study

MOTHER-INFANT INTERACTIONS ARE a cornerstone of early development, supporting social and language development of children with or without autism spectrum disorder (ASD). Research on the impact of maternal behaviors on these interactions offers helpful guidance in clinical work with infants with ASD.

This study looked at the interactions between mothers and infants in families where at least one other child in the family had ASD. These infants are considered to have high risk for ASD. It was a prospective study, having partners rate the mothers using a well-standardized instrument, the Social Responsiveness Scale (SRS), and having trained coders rate videotaped interactions of mothers with the infant. The control group consisted of mothers and infants with no family history of ASD. These control infants are considered to be at low risk for having ASD.

The SRS differentiates well between typically developing (TD), at-risk, and ASD populations. And for the video measure, maternal social behavior in context (during play) was assessed by looking at face, vocalization, and positive affect. All of the infants were assessed using a common autism instrument, the Autism Diagnostic Observation Scale (ADOS), at 36 months of age and classified as ASD, TD, or non-TD.

RESULTS

In both the high- and low-risk infants, mothers had similar responsiveness, not significantly different (p = 0.40), both falling within normal range of reciprocal social behavior (t-scores < 60). These findings held at 6, 9, and 12 months of age. Mothers in the high-risk group used slightly fewer responses than the low-risk group at 9 and 12 months, but these differences were neither statistically nor clinically significant—although in both groups, mothers with boys and mothers from higher-income families tended to talk more to their babies. On the ADOS, all the infants increased their frequency of social behavior responses to their mothers over time, which was good news.

And here's the key finding: In both groups, when mothers had positive emotional tone and tried to find more ways to connect with their children, the infants also had more positive emotions, vocalized more, looked at their mothers more, responded more, and very importantly, initiated more interactions. This pattern was most consistent when infants were 12 months of age.

THE CARLAT TAKE

This study has several clinically relevant findings. The severity of an infant's difficulties did not dissuade the mother's efforts to communicate, infants generally improved with time, and mothers' positive affect and efforts to engage and interact were associated with improved social communication in their infants no matter the severity of the condition.

PRACTICE IMPLICATIONS

These findings underline the importance of encouraging mothers to persist in attempting to engage infants with autism and related challenges. All infants need positive, face-to-face interactions with their mothers—their efforts are likely to bear fruit.

Heart Rate Changes Linked to Emotional Dysregulation

REVIEW OF: Deutz MHF, Woltering S, Vossen HGM, et al. **Underlying psychophysiology of dysregulation: Resting heart rate and heart rate reactivity in relation to childhood dysregulation.** *J Am Acad Child Adolesc Psychiatry.* 2019 Jun;58(6):589–599.

STUDY TYPE: Cross-sectional study

CAN WE USE heart rate to assess and track psychopathology? Child psychiatrists associate lower resting heart rate (HR-rest) and heart rate reactivity (HR-reactivity) with externalizing behaviors such as disruptive behaviors and aggression ("under-arousal") and elevations with internalizing problems such as anxiety ("over-arousal"). The transdiagnostic approach of the NIH Research Diagnostic Criteria (RDoC) offers research linking heart rate with emotional dysregulation. This study bridges these ideas to clinical practice.

In this Canadian study, the authors explored how HR-rest and HR-reactivity relate to dysregulation: 182 clinically referred children (75.8% boys) ages 8–12 years underwent heart rate monitoring at rest and during a computerized go/no-go task. 24.2% of children were on psychotropic medications, mostly stimulants. Dysregulation was measured from subscale scores on the clinically ubiquitous Child Behavior Checklist, specifically the Dysregulation Profile (CBCL-DP), which itself is intricately related to the CBCL Anxious/Depressed, Aggression, and Attention Problems subscales.

RESULTS

These researchers found that higher resting heart rate correlated to higher scores on the dysregulation and aggression subscales, but not to anxiety/depression or attention problems. Heart rate reactivity was not correlated to any of these scales. Although males were more likely to have elevated dysregulation and aggression scores, there was no link between gender and resting heart rate and reactivity.

The researchers also used a person-centered approach, in which subgroups with similar profiles were identified. This approach found that patients tended to sort into three symptom-profile groups: normative (n = 92), predominantly aggressive (n = 69), and dysregulated (n = 14). The dysregulated group had the highest scores (more symptomatic) for anxiety/depression, aggression, and attention problems. When the researchers mapped heart rate parameters onto these profiles, they found that youth in the predominantly aggressive group had higher HR-rest. In contrast, youth in the dysregulated group did not have elevated HR-rest but did have elevated HR-reactivity.

THE CARLAT TAKE

Given the variability among people and confounding variables such as past trauma, it is difficult to apply these findings directly to individual patients. Still, with most of the heart rate literature focused on callous unemotional traits, this study reinforces the importance of looking beyond the categorical descriptors of the DSM and toward a more biologically informed approach.

PRACTICE IMPLICATIONS

One day, perhaps we will be able to use simple physiological measures to help differentiate categories of diagnoses as well as alert us to patients who may have more propensity for aggression. In the future we could be integrating heart rate data into the biopsychosocial model of formulating our patients' diagnoses.

EFFECTS OF CANNABIS

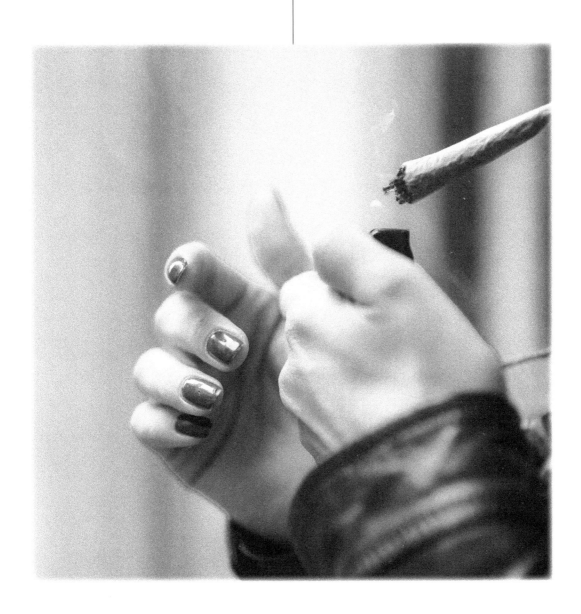

Is There a Case for Cannabis in the Treatment of Pain?

REVIEW OF: **De Vita MJ, Moskal D, Maisto SA, Ansell EB. Association of cannabinoid administration with experimental pain in healthy adults: A systematic review and meta-analysis. *JAMA Psychiatry*. 2018 Nov 1;75(11):1118–1127.**

STUDY TYPE: **Meta-analysis of randomized placebo-controlled trials**

IN THE MIDST of the opioid epidemic, researchers are looking for new ways to treat acute and chronic pain. Interestingly, states that have legalized medical marijuana have fewer opioid prescriptions but no clear reduction in mortality over time (Shover CL et al, *Proc Natl Acad Sci USA* 2019;116(26):12624–12626). Opioid users who smoke marijuana are less likely to drop out of maintenance treatment programs, while benzodiazepine use predicts worse outcomes in this population (Powell D et al, *J Health Econ* 2018;58:29–42; Socías ME et al, *Addiction* 2018;113(12):2250–2258). Could marijuana have direct benefits in the treatment of pain?

To address this question, researchers analyzed 18 placebo-controlled trials of cannabinoids as a treatment for mechanically induced pain in otherwise healthy subjects. For this study of acute pain threshold and tolerance, those with chronic pain were excluded. A total of 442 participants were included. Mean age was 27 with equal numbers of men and women. Two-thirds of the studies involved synthetic tetrahydrocannabinol (THC), the cannabinoid responsible for the "high" in marijuana, or controlled prescription-only analogues of THC, such as dronabinol (C-III) and nabilone (C-II). The other third used plant-based cannabis. The majority (89%) used a crossover design where subjects received both cannabinoids and placebo with a washout period between the doses.

RESULTS

Compared to placebo, cannabinoid administration was associated with a small increase in pain threshold and a small-to-medium increase in pain tolerance. However, it did not change overall pain intensity. Cannabinoids made people better able to withstand a greater pain burden, but only to a certain point. They also made the experience of pain less unpleasant (small-to-medium effect size), and this effect was strongest with plant-based cannabis. *Unpleasantness* is important because it may influence the progression from chronic pain to depression. No significant association was found between cannabinoid administration and hypersensitivity to pain. Gender did not significantly impact any of the outcomes.

THE CARLAT TAKE

The biggest limitation to the study is the lack of blinding as most subjects could probably guess whether or not they were "high." Furthermore, it is unclear how well mechanically induced pain approximates real, chronic pain. Lastly, cannabidiol (CBD) was not included in the study. CBD is often praised by enthusiasts for its properties and was recently approved as prescription Epidiolex for intractable seizures. Unlike THC, CBD produces no "high" and may have added antipsychotic effects.

PRACTICE IMPLICATIONS

Despite the widespread use of THC for a variety of ailments, little data exist to support its many claimed benefits. Additionally, the risks, including psychosis, are too large to recommend it to patients as an alternative analgesic.

Is Cannabis Bad for Cognition?

REVIEW OF: Scott JC, Slomiak ST, Jones JD, et al. **Association of cannabis with cognitive functioning in adolescents and young adults: A systematic review and meta-analysis.** *JAMA Psychiatry.* 2018 Jun 1;75(6):585–595.

STUDY TYPE: **Meta-analysis of observational studies**

OUR PATIENTS TYPICALLY tell us that, according to the internet, weed is perfectly safe and does not affect their ability to think or function. At least 30 states and the District of Columbia have laws legalizing cannabis, supporting the notion that people have begun to think of marijuana as relatively harmless. Rates of marijuana use in young adults are rising (Hasin DS, *Neuropsychopharmacology* 2018;43(1):195–212). Moreover, a recent study reported that cannabidiol (CBD), a "non-psychoactive" component of marijuana, may reduce psychotic symptoms (Arain M et al, *Neuropsychiatr Dis Treat* 2013;9:449–461).

Given that the brain continues to develop into a person's mid-20s, how dangerous is marijuana use in adolescence and young adulthood? And what do we tell our young patients who are regular users? A new meta-analysis attempts to answer part of that question as it relates to the impact of cannabis use on cognitive function in adolescents and young adults.

RESULTS

The meta-analysis assessed cognitive effects in young adults and adolescents whose primary clinical problem was cannabis use. The analysis included 69 studies of 2,152 regular cannabis users and 6,575 people with minimal use of cannabis. After combining the results from all of these studies, the authors concluded that cannabis does have a mild negative correlation with various aspects of cognition. Specifically, studies showed that use of the drug is negatively associated with executive functioning, speed of information processing, delayed memory, working memory, and attention. But in the aggregate, effect sizes range from −0.21 to −0.33, indicating minimal impact on cognition. Verbal language, visuospatial functioning, and motor functioning were relatively spared. Studies that required at least 72 hours of cannabis abstinence before testing reported no significant effect on cognitive function.

THE CARLAT TAKE

At first glance, these results may seem reassuring. Cognition was minimally impacted, and the effects did not extend beyond active use. However, many of the studies were small, measurement of cannabis use and potency varied, and significant publication bias was noted. Also, the meta-analysis focused solely on neurocognitive effects and ignored other clinically pertinent outcomes.

PRACTICE IMPLICATIONS

Another study looking at 3,826 seventh graders found neurotoxic effects of cannabis on memory and inhibitory control (Morin JG et al, *Am J Psychiatry* 2019;176(2):98–106). Moreover, we have ample evidence that marijuana use is associated with poor academic and social function, that the tetrahydrocannabinol (THC) component of marijuana is associated with an overall doubling of psychosis risk in youth, and that this increased psychosis risk is dose dependent. So, however you interpret this analysis, THC is clearly not off the hook.

Effects of Cannabis Use on Smoking Cessation

REVIEW OF: Weinberger AH, Platt J, Copeland J, Goodwin RD. Is cannabis use associated with increased risk of cigarette smoking initiation, persistence, and relapse? Longitudinal data from a representative sample of US adults. *J Clin Psychiatry*. 2018 Mar/Apr;79(2):17m11522.

STUDY TYPE: Prospective cohort study

WHEN COUNSELING YOUR patients to quit smoking, you may also want to consider asking them about their past marijuana use. Results from a recent study suggest that there may be a correlation between cannabis and tobacco smoking.

Analysis of longitudinal data of almost 35,000 adult study participants, gathered during two "waves" (2001–2002 and 2004–2005) of the US National Epidemiologic Survey on Alcohol and Related Conditions, found that past cannabis use was associated with an increase in cigarette smoking initiation, persistence, and relapse.

RESULTS

In the study, cannabis use was associated with a 2.9-fold and 4.4-fold increased risk of new cigarette use on either a daily or non-daily basis, respectively, compared to those without exposure to cannabis in the previous year. Among former smokers, past cannabis use was associated with increased relapse rate: 4.18 times more ex-smokers returned to daily smoking and 5.24 times more ex-smokers returned to smoking on a non-daily basis compared to those who had not used cannabinoids in the past 12 months.

Past cannabis use was also associated with difficulty quitting tobacco: Among daily cigarette smokers, past cannabinoid use was associated with decreased odds of smoking cessation by 43% compared with non-cannabis users. Even when demographics and a history of psychiatric disorders were taken into consideration, associations of cannabis use remained significant for the initiation of daily smoking among prior nonsmokers; relapsing to a daily use pattern among former ex-smokers; and difficulty quitting among daily smokers.

THE CARLAT TAKE

This study provides some interesting data showing that people who use cannabis are more likely to start smoking tobacco. Cannabis use was also associated in more difficulty quitting smoking and more likely return to smoking for ex-smokers.

PRACTICE IMPLICATIONS

Tell your patients that if they've used cannabis in the past, quitting tobacco may be more of a challenge than usual. This will set the stage for a discussion of the various smoking cessation agents available, and it might increase your patients' motivation to accept treatment.

Can Computerized Interventions Reduce Cannabis Use?

REVIEW OF: Olmos A, Tirado-Muñoz J, Farré M, Torrens M. The efficacy of computerized interventions to reduce cannabis use: A systematic review and meta-analysis. *Addict Behav*. 2018 Apr;79:52–60.

STUDY TYPE: Systematic review and meta-analysis

As medical and recreational marijuana become legalized in more states, more emphasis is being placed on treatment of those with cannabis use disorders. But with our clinics already at capacity, how can we find the most efficient way of providing therapy? Computerized interventions are already available for nicotine and alcohol use, but what about for cannabis?

This meta-analysis included nine randomized controlled trials evaluating the efficacy of web-based treatments designed to reduce the frequency of cannabis use. The primary outcome was reduction in cannabis use, and the secondary outcome was reduction in other substance use. A total of 2,963 participants were included in the studies—1,724 in the intervention groups and 1,239 in the control groups. All the interventions were computer based, and the control conditions varied from study to study—from no intervention to psychoeducation.

RESULTS

So, how did the computer-based interventions fare? Those who participated in the computerized interventions had a significant reduction in cannabis use when compared to the control groups (SMD: −0.19; 95% CI: −0.26 to −0.11), with no significant heterogeneity among the studies (I2 = 0%). Only three of the nine trials collected data on the secondary outcome of reduction in other substance use, but there was again a significant reduction in those studies compared to the control condition (SMD: −0.27; 95% CI: −0.46 to −0.08), with low heterogeneity (I2 = 26%). Several sub-group analyses were performed, but the only significant result was in the number of sessions—interventions with ≥ 5 sessions performed better than those with < 5 sessions (SMD: −0.21; 95% CI −0.29 to −0.12).

THE CARLAT TAKE

With more people seeking treatment for substance use disorders, we need more options to give them effective care. This analysis shows that computerized interventions can work to help patients reduce cannabis use, along with other substance use. But the verdict is still out on web-based interventions. A more recent Swedish study showed no effect on cannabis use for a web-based treatment program with therapist guidance versus a waitlist control group (Sinadinovic K et al, *Addict Sci Clin Pract* 2020;15(1):9).

PRACTICE IMPLICATIONS

When considering computer-based interventions, it's also important to note what the study doesn't show: There was no comparison to a live therapist intervention. Sessions with an in-person therapist are still recommended, but when that's not available, offering a computer-based intervention may be a good option.

OPIOID USE DISORDER

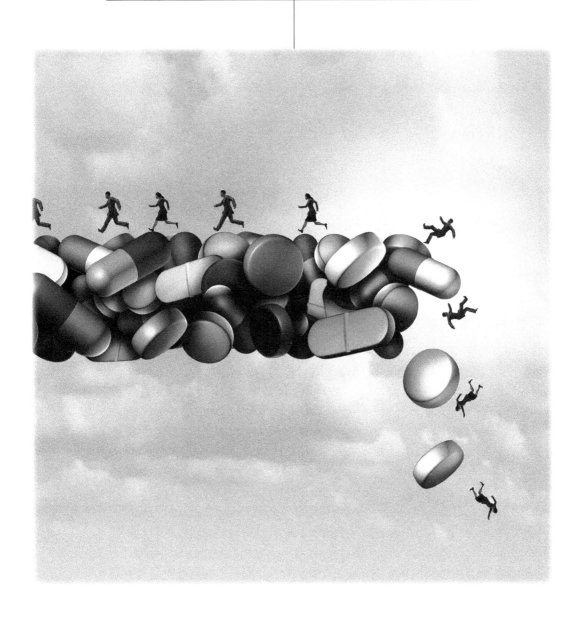

Oral vs Extended-Release Naltrexone for Opioid Use Disorder

REVIEW OF: **Sullivan M, Bisaga A, Pavlicova M, et al. Long-acting injectable naltrexone induction: A randomized trial of outpatient opioid detoxification with naltrexone versus buprenorphine.** *Am J Psychiatry.* **2017 May 1;174(5):459–467.**

STUDY TYPE: **Randomized, open-label trial**

EXTENDED-RELEASE (XR) NALTREXONE (Vivitrol) is FDA approved for opioid use disorder (OUD) and has shown efficacy in several trials. It works best for patients who have already successfully detoxed from opioids and who are highly motivated to abstain. But what about oral naltrexone? While it is effective for alcohol use disorder, studies for OUD have shown limited utility. The reason is obvious—patients who are experiencing high cravings can simply skip a dose of the naltrexone pill in order to achieve an opioid high, whereas the XR formulation forces a long delay, during which patients might reconsider their decision to use. Oddly enough, though, no study has been done comparing oral to XR naltrexone, until now.

Researchers randomized 60 adults with OUD (DSM-IV opioid dependence) to either oral or XR naltrexone. The study was a 6-month open-label trial, excluding people with unstable medical or psychiatric disorders, physical dependence on alcohol or sedative-hypnotics, treatment with opioids or psychotropic medications, and history of opioid overdose in the prior 3 years. The primary outcome measure was retention in treatment.

The study didn't quite mimic real-world treatment, as study participants in both groups were asked to attend behavioral therapy sessions twice weekly, and those randomized to oral naltrexone either had to have a responsible adult as an involved medication monitor at home or go to the clinic 3 times weekly to have it administered. Vouchers were used to reinforce attendance. Participants were mostly white (63.3%), male (83.3%), and in their late 30s (mean age 39.5, SD = 11.1).

RESULTS

At the end of 6 months, the retention rate in the XR naltrexone group was significantly higher than the oral naltrexone group (57.1% and 28.1%, respectively). There was no significant difference in the percentage of opioid-positive urine tests between the groups, though that was not the primary outcome, and missed urine tests were not counted as positive. Overall, the treatment was well tolerated, and most adverse events reflected opioid withdrawal and gradually improved.

THE CARLAT TAKE

The results confirm that XR naltrexone is more effective than oral naltrexone for OUD, even when rigorous strategies are used to ensure adherence with the oral formulation. However, oral naltrexone still has its place in treating alcohol use disorder.

PRACTICE IMPLICATIONS

When treating OUD, use oral naltrexone to test tolerance and sensitivity before transitioning to XR naltrexone. We still recommend reserving XR naltrexone for patients who cannot be on buprenorphine or methadone—medications for which we have even more robust data.

Does Extended-Release Naltrexone Worsen Psychiatric Symptoms?

REVIEW OF: Latif ZEH, Benth JŠ, Solli KK, et al. Anxiety, depression, and insomnia among adults with opioid dependence treated with extended-release naltrexone vs buprenorphine-naloxone: A randomized clinical trial and follow-up study. *JAMA Psychiatry*. 2019 Feb 1;76(2):127–134.

STUDY TYPE: Randomized, single-blind, active-controlled trial

EXTENDED-RELEASE (XR) NALTREXONE (Vivitrol) is an injectable version of naltrexone that lasts for 4 weeks and is FDA approved for opioid use disorder (OUD). Although effective, there is some concern that XR naltrexone may cause or worsen psychiatric symptoms because of its opioid blockade. Prior research has been mixed on this issue, and studies have been limited by not comparing XR naltrexone with an active control medication. This new study is the first to directly compare XR naltrexone with buprenorphine in terms of their effects on anxiety, depression, and insomnia.

The outpatient Norwegian study contained two components: a 12-week randomized controlled trial (RCT) and a 36-week follow-up study. In the RCT, 159 participants diagnosed with OUD were randomly assigned, but not blinded, to treatment with flexibly dosed daily buprenorphine/naloxone or monthly injections of XR naltrexone. At the end of 12 weeks, participants could choose treatment with buprenorphine/naloxone or XR naltrexone, and they were then followed for an additional 36 weeks.

Outcome measures included symptoms of anxiety, depression, and insomnia, as assessed by the Hopkins Symptom Checklist and the Insomnia Severity Index. These scales measure symptoms, but they are not diagnostic, and there was no mention of the prevalence and distribution of mood, anxiety, and sleep disorders between the groups.

RESULTS

The results showed that the two treatments were comparable. During the RCT component of this study, XR naltrexone was not significantly different than buprenorphine in terms of anxiety and depression symptoms, and it was slightly better than buprenorphine regarding insomnia symptoms (effect size −0.32; p = 0.008). There were no significant differences between groups in the follow-up component. Encouragingly, throughout all components of the study, anxiety, depression, and insomnia symptoms improved over time.

THE CARLAT TAKE

It appears that XR naltrexone does not worsen symptoms of anxiety, depression, or insomnia in people with OUD and even improved throughout the study. Strengths of the study include long follow-up time and real-world design in the open-label extension period.

PRACTICE IMPLICATIONS

When we are deciding between XR naltrexone and buprenorphine/naloxone for OUD, the primary factors should be efficacy and patient access and preference. Both medications are effective in treating OUD and according to this research would not exacerbate psychiatric symptoms.

Switching From Buprenorphine to Extended-Release Naltrexone: Does It Work?

REVIEW OF: **Solli KK, Latif ZEH, Opheim A, et al. Effectiveness, safety and feasibility of extended-release naltrexone for opioid dependence: A 9-month follow-up to a 3-month randomized trial. *Addiction*. 2018 Oct;113(10):1840–1849.**

STUDY TYPE: **Prospective cohort study**

EXTENDED-RELEASE (XR) NALTREXONE (Vivitrol) has had some good data, yet getting patients on it remains a challenge because an opioid-free period is required before starting it. Understandably, practitioners get nervous when patients stabilized on buprenorphine ask to be transitioned to XR naltrexone. But if needed, can this switch be made safely and effectively?

To answer this question, researchers in Norway conducted an open-label continuation of a 3-month controlled trial (see "Does Extended-Release Naltrexone Worsen Psychiatric Symptoms?" on the previous page). In the original study, 159 patients were randomized to up to 24 mg of buprenorphine/ naloxone daily or 380 mg of XR naltrexone injection monthly. At the end of 3 months, participants were offered the option of continuing on XR naltrexone, switching from buprenorphine to XR naltrexone, or treatment with buprenorphine at a program outside the study. Of the 122 participants who completed the first phase, 117 chose XR naltrexone, and 5 chose buprenorphine outside of the study. XR naltrexone was not commercially available in Norway, which may account for the large number of people choosing it over buprenorphine.

The switch was carefully made during a detox admission, where XR naltrexone was initiated after a test dose of naloxone and a minimum of 72 hours following any opioid intake (which is a lot shorter than the commonly recommended washout period), and adjunctive medications were available to help relieve withdrawal symptoms. Participants were followed for another 9 months, and the primary outcomes were continuation of treatment and abstinence rates for those who remained on XR naltrexone (n = 54) compared with those who switched to XR naltrexone (n = 63).

Participants were men and women ages 18–60 years with opioid use disorder (DSM-IV opioid dependence) and without alcohol dependence or serious somatic or psychiatric comorbidities. Pregnant and nursing women were excluded. The majority of participants were men (75%), and the mean age was 35.6 years.

RESULTS

Nine months later, there were no significant differences in outcomes between participants who continued XR naltrexone and those who switched to it from buprenorphine. Twenty-eight participants (51.9%) who were originally on XR naltrexone and 30 (47.6%) who newly started on it completed 9 months of follow-up. Complete abstinence from opioids was self-reported by 53.7% of participants continuing XR naltrexone and 44.4% of those newly started. Adverse events were generally related to withdrawal symptoms. Two patients discontinued XR naltrexone due to serious injection site reactions requiring surgery, after which they recovered completely.

THE CARLAT TAKE

The results of the study imply that switching from buprenorphine to XR naltrexone may work as well as starting XR naltrexone from scratch. The study was not perfect—the design was open-label, there was no objective confirmation of abstinence, and the switch was carefully done on an inpatient unit, limiting our confidence that it can be done as safely and effectively in outpatient settings.

PRACTICE IMPLICATIONS

The naturalistic setting of this study makes it similar to clinical practice, and the 50% self-reported abstinence rate is encouraging. Switching from buprenorphine to XR naltrexone can be attempted in select patients, but we recommend approaching switch requests with great caution. We continue to think of XR naltrexone as a second-line option for patients who cannot be on agonist treatment.

More Evidence of Lives Saved by Medications for Opioid Use Disorder

REVIEW OF: Larochelle MR, Bernson D, Land T, et al. Medication for opioid use disorder after nonfatal opioid overdose and association with mortality: A cohort study. *Ann Intern Med.* 2018 Aug 7;169(3):137–145.

STUDY TYPE: Retrospective cohort study

WE ARE IN the middle of an opioid crisis in the US, with many lives lost daily to opioid-related deaths. Pharmacotherapy with methadone, buprenorphine, or naltrexone represents an important tool for clinicians during this crisis. But just how good are these medications in saving lives? A recent retrospective cohort study evaluated the effects of methadone, buprenorphine, and naltrexone on all-cause and opioid-related mortality in the 12 months after an opioid overdose.

This analysis used data from Massachusetts government and hospital records from 2012 to 2014 to identify adults who survived an opioid overdose, then looked at the 12 months after that overdose. If an individual had multiple overdoses during that period, the first overdose was used for the data collection. A total of 17,568 cases were identified. In the 12 months after the index overdose, 11% (2,040) were on methadone for a median of 5 months, 17% (3,022) were on buprenorphine for a median of 4 months, and 6% (1,099) were on naltrexone for a median of 1 month.

RESULTS

All-cause mortality over 12 months was significantly reduced in those receiving methadone (adjusted hazard ratio [AHR] 0.47 [CI 0.32–0.71]) and buprenorphine (AHR 0.63 [CI 0.46–0.87]), but not those on naltrexone (AHR 1.44 [CI 0.84–2.46]). Similarly, opioid-related mortality was significantly decreased for patients on methadone (AHR 0.41 [CI 0.24–0.70]) and buprenorphine (AHR 0.62 [CI 0.41–0.92]), but not those on naltrexone (AHR 1.42 [CI 0.73–2.79]).

THE CARLAT TAKE

This study represents real-world population data linking treatment with methadone or buprenorphine after an opioid overdose to a decrease in all-cause and opioid-related mortality in the following year. Remember, these results were tallied over a 1-year period even though most patients discontinued treatment within 6 months. Naltrexone failed to show a significant difference in mortality, perhaps because most people stopped it after 1 month, or because the researchers could not distinguish between the oral and extended-release injectable formulations (unlike oral naltrexone, extended-release naltrexone has shown treatment efficacy).

PRACTICE IMPLICATIONS

Another takeaway from this article is that only about a third of those who had an opioid overdose were ever prescribed any form of opioid use disorder pharmacotherapy. More lives could be saved with medication-assisted treatment. Much work remains to be done to provide better access to life-saving treatment for opioid use disorder.

Guidelines for Switching From Methadone to Buprenorphine

REVIEW OF: Lintzeris N, Monds LA, Rivas C, et al. Transferring patients from methadone to buprenorphine: The feasibility and evaluation of practice guidelines. *J Addict Med.* **2018 May/Jun;12(3):234–240.**

STUDY TYPE: Prospective cohort study

RECENT GUIDELINES PUBLISHED by the American Society of Addiction Medicine (ASAM) and nationally in Australia provide support for transferring patients from methadone to buprenorphine/naloxone (BNX). Patients may switch thinking BNX is easier to discontinue or because of methadone side effects. The transition can be complicated by relapses or precipitated withdrawal when starting BNX. To minimize adverse events, the ASAM and Australian guidelines recommend the following (summarized; Kampman K and Jarvis M, *J Addict Med* 2015;9(5):358–367):

1. Consider inpatient treatment for patients with significant medical comorbidities, with unstable social conditions, or transferring from high methadone doses (> 50 mg/day).

2. Gradually reduce methadone until the patient experiences mild to moderate opioid withdrawal symptoms between doses.

3. Stop methadone and begin monitoring regularly for opioid withdrawal, using measures such as the Clinical Opiate Withdrawal Scale (COWS).

4. Start low-dose BNX at 2 mg, at least 24 hours after the last dose of methadone and after the patient experiences moderate opioid withdrawal (COWS score > 12), monitoring hourly afterwards for precipitated withdrawal.

5. Administer 6 mg after 1 hour; additional doses, 4–8 mg, are symptom triggered.

6. On successive days: BNX dosage = the previous day's dose plus additional symptom-triggered doses.

Lintzeris and colleagues studied the clinical feasibility of these guidelines. They reviewed medical records of four Australian specialist addiction centers to assess the outcomes of guideline feasibility, transfer practices, and patient responses.

RESULTS

In all, 33 adult participants transferred, 9 from low-dose (LD) methadone (< 30 mg/day), 9 from medium-dose (MD) methadone (30–50 mg/day), and 15 from high-dose (HD) methadone (> 50 mg/day). Most HD transfers occurred in inpatient settings (93%), while most MD/LD transfers occurred in outpatient settings (67%). Inpatient stays were 2.2 days on average. 70% of transfers were consistent with the guidelines. Most patients stabilized their BNX dose by day 3, with 96% using ≥ 12 mg/day. Overall, 79% (26/33) were still on BNX treatment at day 7 and were considered to have successfully transferred.

Three patients experienced precipitated withdrawal, all in the HD group, and all returning to methadone. Three patients resumed methadone due to anxiety and poor sleep with BNX. One participant relapsed and used heroin for several days before resuming methadone.

THE CARLAT TAKE

Although this was a small sample, the findings are useful. They suggest most patients can successfully transfer from methadone to BNX when using the guidelines. Those transferring from HD methadone require inpatient settings and specialist supervision, while most MD/LD methadone transfers may be suitable for outpatient clinics. It is important to avoid precipitated withdrawal, as that will most likely lead to failed transfer to BNX.

PRACTICE IMPLICATIONS

These guidelines are easy to follow and provide practical advice on how to transition from methadone to BNX. Close monitoring during the initial test doses of BNX is paramount. If followed, precipitated withdrawal is unlikely to happen, and most patients will be able to successfully transition to BNX.

Opioids Not Superior to Other Medicines for Some Chronic Pain

REVIEW OF: Krebs EE, Gravely A, Nugent S, et al. Effect of opioid vs nonopioid medications on pain-related function in patients with chronic back pain or hip or knee osteoarthritis pain: The SPACE randomized clinical trial. *JAMA*. 2018 Mar 6;319(9):872–882.

STUDY TYPE: Randomized, single-blind, active-controlled trial

RISING RATES OF opioid overdose deaths have sounded alarm bells over opioid prescribing practices for chronic pain. Unfortunately, and despite the absence of quality data on risks vs benefits, long-term opioid management has remained a common approach to managing chronic musculoskeletal pain.

This study examined long-term outcomes in chronic pain with opioid vs non-opioid treatment. Researchers conducted a 12-month randomized trial evaluating patients who—despite analgesic use—had moderate to severe chronic back pain or hip/knee osteoarthritic pain. Patients were recruited from Veterans Affairs primary care clinics in Minneapolis, Minnesota between 2013 and 2015.

The study compared opioid and non-opioid therapy. Patients in each group were prescribed multiple medications over three steps. In total, 240 patients were randomized, with a mean age of 58.3 years; females made up 13% of the group.

In the opioid group, the first phase was immediate-release morphine, oxycodone, or hydrocodone/acetaminophen. Second- and third-step options included sustained-action morphine and transdermal fentanyl.

For the non-opioid group, the first stage was acetaminophen or an NSAID. Second- and third-phase choices comprised adjuvants, such as gabapentin or nortriptyline; topical analgesics; and drugs such as duloxetine and tramadol.

Outcomes measured included the impact of pain on daily functioning, rated on the Brief Pain Inventory [BPI] interference scale; pain intensity on the BPI severity scale; and adverse medication-related symptoms. The BPI interference scale records the influence of pain on activities like sleep, walking, relationships, work, and life enjoyment. For both BPI scales, the range is 0–10, with higher scores indicating worsened functioning or higher pain intensity.

RESULTS

Over 12 months, the groups did not significantly differ on pain-related function. The mean BPI interference was 3.4 for the opioid group and 3.3 for the non-opioid group. Unexpectedly, the non-opioid group reported significantly less pain intensity at 12 months, with a BPI severity of 4.0 for the opioid group and 3.5 for the non-opioid group. Adverse medication-related symptoms were significantly more common in the opioid group.

THE CARLAT TAKE

The noteworthy result here is that chronic pain patients on opioids may not be any better off than those taking alternative agents. While psychiatrists are not the primary treaters of musculoskeletal pain, the current opioid crisis has had wide-ranging impact, and there are calls for a multipronged approach.

PRACTICE IMPLICATIONS

Many patients with chronic pain develop opioid dependence after long-term opioid treatment, and we should be ready to share this study's results with our patients and medical colleagues. There are a variety of non-opioid medication treatments that may not only treat chronic pain but have less long-term side effects or risks overall.

ALCOHOL USE DISORDER

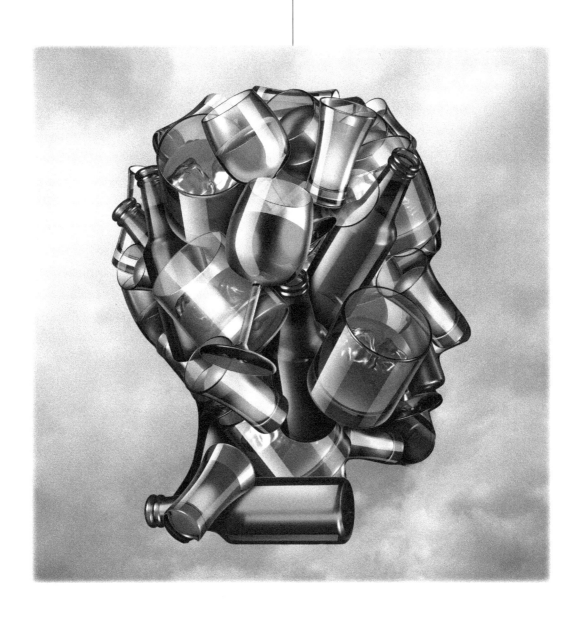

Prazosin for Alcohol Use Disorder

REVIEW OF: Simpson TL, Saxon AJ, Stappenbeck C, et al. Double-blind randomized clinical trial of prazosin for alcohol use disorder. *Am J Psychiatry*. 2018 Dec 1;175(12):1216–1224.

STUDY TYPE: Randomized, double-blind, placebo-controlled trial

Prazosin is often used as a second-line option for a broad array of psychiatric conditions, including anxiety, insomnia, nightmares, and post-traumatic stress disorder (PTSD). It is a high blood pressure medication that also modulates the stress-response system through noradrenergic effects, blocking alpha-1 receptors in the brain. Since stress is a common trigger for excessive drinking, this study set out to test whether prazosin could improve sobriety in alcohol use disorder (AUD).

Eighty subjects with AUD were randomized to receive either prazosin or placebo. Subjects with PTSD were excluded in order to isolate the potential benefits of prazosin for drinking directly. Prazosin was titrated up to a target dosage of 16 mg/day, as tolerated. All subjects were actively drinking at the start of the study, and they reported their daily alcohol consumption and cravings for the previous day through a toll-free interactive voice system during the 12-week study. Assessments were double-blind, and the primary outcomes were number of drinks per week, number of drinking days per week, and number of heavy drinking days per week.

RESULTS

Compared to placebo, those receiving prazosin reported fewer drinks (mean decrease of 8.0 vs 1.5 drinks per week; p = 0.03) and fewer heavy drinking days (mean decrease of 0.8 vs 0.3 days per week; p = 0.01), though the number of drinking days was no less with prazosin. Drowsiness and edema were the only two side effects associated with prazosin.

THE CARLAT TAKE

This trial gives us some encouraging evidence that prazosin can help people reduce their drinking. We know that for those with AUD, any decrease in the amount someone is drinking can lead to better health outcomes. Other studies have shown limited efficacy of prazosin for AUD, but on post-hoc analysis it may be more helpful for those with higher drinks per week at baseline (Wilcox CE et al, *J Addict Med* 2018;12(5):339–345).

PRACTICE IMPLICATIONS

Given its relatively benign side effect profile and established track record, prazosin can be considered a reasonable second-line option for AUD. For patients with any combination of anxiety, insomnia, nightmares, PTSD, or hypertension, prazosin is an even more appealing option.

The COMBINE Study: A Core Paper in the Treatment of AUD

REVIEW OF: Anton RF, O'Malley SS, Ciraulo DA, et al. Combined pharmacotherapies and behavioral interventions for alcohol dependence: The COMBINE study: A randomized controlled trial. *JAMA*. 2006 May 3;295(17):2003–2017.

STUDY TYPE: Randomized, single-blind, placebo-controlled trial

CONDUCTED FROM 2001 to 2004 and published in 2006, the COMBINE study was the largest pharmacotherapy study that assessed the treatment of alcohol use disorder (AUD). Although there were significant data on the use of naltrexone and acamprosate (both had been FDA approved), widespread use had not been adopted for either medication, and extended-release naltrexone was still undergoing its approval process. The prior large NIAAA-funded study of AUD interventions was Project MATCH, which focused exclusively on psychosocial therapies, whereas COMBINE evaluated the effectiveness of naltrexone, acamprosate, and specialty therapy both alone and in combination. By doing so, the authors hoped to shed light on the following questions: 1) Are there synergistic intervention combinations? 2) Is effective treatment of AUD feasible in a primary care setting?

A total of 1,383 recently abstinent subjects across 11 academic sites were randomly assigned to nine groups, and the trial was conducted over 16 weeks. Outcomes included percentage of days abstinent and return to heavy drinking. Combined behavioral intervention (CBI), an amalgamation of the evidence-based therapies used in Project MATCH (cognitive behavioral therapy, 12-step facilitation, and motivational interviewing), was a specialty therapy developed for this study. One group received only CBI (no pills) and the eight pill-taking groups received varying combinations of CBI, acamprosate, naltrexone, and placebo, including a placebo-only group. Those eight groups also received medical management (MM), a brief evaluative and supportive intervention with a health care professional similar to a primary care encounter.

RESULTS

Compared to placebo, naltrexone reduced the percentage of participants who returned to heavy drinking (68.2% vs 71.4%; p = 0.02), but not percentage of days abstinent (78.8% vs 77.2%; p = 0.25). In contrast, acamprosate did not separate from placebo in any condition or interaction. A more striking result, however, was how poorly the CBI-only group performed in comparison to the pill-taking + MM groups, including in comparison to the placebo groups. For instance, placebo groups produced significantly greater percentage of days abstinent than CBI alone (p < 0.001). Although the authors point out a statistically significant interaction between CBI and naltrexone, this is not very convincing, as the data for this interaction included subjects receiving placebo. For those who received actual naltrexone, the CBI + naltrexone group was no better than naltrexone alone.

THE CARLAT TAKE

This core study of AUD treatment is worth looking at again as it has guided our clinical decision-making. Strengths include a large number of participants and treatment sites, which allowed for many comparison arms. This study emphasized primary care settings and not needing specialty referral to access initial medication management for AUD.

PRACTICE IMPLICATIONS

This study demonstrates that evidence-based AUD treatment can be delivered in non-specialty settings, which would expand access tremendously. Although clearly not a panacea, naltrexone performed well in the MM model. Acamprosate did not fare well, and it may perform better when initiated after a longer period of abstinence. This was also a disappointing study for psychotherapy, but the findings aren't enough reason to write it off, and psychosocial interventions in addiction treatment continue to be a recommended part of the treatment plan.

Gabapentin Enacarbil XR Efficacy Less Than Expected for AUD

REVIEW OF: Falk DE, Ryan ML, Fertig JB, et al. Gabapentin enacarbil extended-release for alcohol use disorder: A randomized, double-blind, placebo-controlled, multisite trial assessing efficacy and safety. *Alcohol Clin Exp Res.* 2019 Jan;43(1):158–169.

STUDY TYPE: Randomized, double-blind, placebo-controlled trial

GABAPENTIN ENACARBIL EXTENDED-RELEASE (GE-XR) (Horizant) is an extended-release version of gabapentin. GE-XR is a prodrug, meaning that once ingested it is metabolized into gabapentin. It is currently approved for treatment of postherpetic neuralgia and restless legs syndrome. It differs from the immediate-release (IR) version in dosing (twice a day for the GE-XR, as opposed to 3 times a day) and has less variable blood levels. Several previous studies showed that IR gabapentin may be helpful for reducing withdrawal symptoms and promoting abstinence in alcohol use disorder (AUD) (Anton RF et al, *Am J Psychiatry* 2011;168(7):709–717; Mason BJ et al, *JAMA Intern Med* 2014;174(1):70–77). Since an extended-release version might be easier to prescribe and increase adherence, researchers tested this XR formulation for AUD.

This trial assigned 346 adults with moderate AUD to two groups: the treatment group (n = 173) received GE-XR tablets titrated to 600 mg twice daily, whereas the control group (also n = 173) received identical placebo tablets. Moderate AUD was defined as ingestion of at least 21 standard drinks per week for women and at least 28 standard drinks per week for men (1 standard drink = 0.6 oz of pure alcohol). Participants were not currently using any other substances and were not diagnosed with a major psychiatric disorder. The trial lasted 26 weeks.

RESULTS

The primary outcome was change in the percentage of subjects with no heavy drinking days, defined as 4 or more drinks for women or 5 or more drinks for men per drinking day. There were several secondary outcomes, such as percentage of heavy drinking days, percentage of days abstinent, and others. For the primary outcome and all secondary outcomes, no statistical advantage was seen between the GE-XR group and placebo. Patients taking GE-XR actually did significantly worse than the placebo group in two of the secondary outcomes: average number of DSM-5 AUD criteria (3.4 vs 2.8; p = 0.046) and depressive symptoms on the Beck Depression Inventory-II (6.5 vs 5.2; p = 0.046).

For the safety assessment, patients in the GE-XR group reported significantly more fatigue (25.9%), somnolence (17.6%), and tremor (5.9%) than the placebo group. There were also more patients reporting suicidal ideation in the GE-XR group (7 vs 1, but just below significance level at p = 0.067).

THE CARLAT TAKE

This study had a strong design, adequate sample size, and a basis for success in the previous positive trials of IR gabapentin (Mason BJ et al, *JAMA Intern Med* 2014;174(1):70–77). However, GE-XR didn't show any positive outcomes and even had worse outcomes for AUD and depressive symptoms.

PRACTICE IMPLICATIONS

These negative findings may have potentially been due to the dosing used in this trial or altered bioavailability of the XR prodrug formulation in an AUD population. Similar trials with IR gabapentin used a higher effective dose. Regardless, GE-XR at the dose studied in this trial can't be recommended for treating AUD at this time.

Prevalence of Fetal Alcohol Spectrum Disorder

REVIEW OF: **May PA, Chambers CD, Kalberg WO, et al. Prevalence of fetal alcohol spectrum disorders in 4 US communities. _JAMA_. 2018 Feb 6;319(5):474–482.**

STUDY TYPE: **Cross-sectional study**

NEW EVIDENCE SUGGESTS that the prevalence of fetal alcohol spectrum disorder is higher than previously documented. In this study, prevalence estimates were derived from 13,146 first-grade children in four US communities between 2010 and 2016.

The study used active-case ascertainment, which the authors assert is a more reliable approach for identifying this cluster of disorders (eg, fetal alcohol syndrome, partial fetal alcohol syndrome, and alcohol-related neurodevelopment disorder). With active-case ascertainment, surveillance personnel conduct research by reviewing data from all areas of a hospital that come in contact with a neonate, instead of limiting themselves to the neonatal intensive care and labor and delivery units.

Furthermore, standardized consensus criteria were employed to classify cases (https://www.cdc.gov/ncbddd/fasd/facts.html). Assessments included four relevant domains: growth, dysmorphology, neurodevelopment, and prenatal alcohol exposure (the latter assessed during maternal interviews).

RESULTS

During this time period, 222 children were identified as having fetal alcohol spectrum disorder. Notably, only 2 of these children had been previously diagnosed. Using the more conservative approach, the prevalence rates of fetal alcohol spectrum disorders across the four sites ranged from 11.3 (95% CI, 7.8–15.8) to 50.0 (95% CI, 39.9–61.7) per 1,000 children. This corresponds to a range of approximately 1%–5%, the latter of which is higher than previous published estimates (eg, 1%–2%). The less conservative estimates that were reported in this study peaked at 98.5 per 1,000 children (nearly 10%) at one site.

THE CARLAT TAKE

According to this new research, fetal alcohol spectrum disorders are not rare events in the US, which suggests we need to improve our ability to detect these cases.

PRACTICE IMPLICATIONS

Given the negative (and preventable) consequences associated with fetal alcohol spectrum disorders (eg, poor academic achievement, mental health disorders), we recommend proactive education on the adverse consequences of drinking alcohol during pregnancy, in addition to enhanced prevention and intervention efforts. Also, support services should be provided for individuals affected by this condition, with the goal of improving their long-term prognosis and enhancing their quality of life.

Is Varenicline Effective for Alcohol Use Disorder?

REVIEW OF: O'Malley SS, Zweben A, Fucito LM, et al. Effect of varenicline combined with medical management on alcohol use disorder with comorbid cigarette smoking: A randomized clinical trial. *JAMA Psychiatry*. 2018 Feb 1;75(2):129–138.

STUDY TYPE: Randomized, double-blind, placebo-controlled trial

ACTING ON THE nicotinic acetylcholine receptors, varenicline (Chantix) is an FDA-approved treatment for smoking cessation. These receptors are implicated in both nicotine and alcohol reward pathways, so could varenicline also be helpful for treating alcohol use disorder (AUD)? So far, the evidence has been mixed, but some studies have shown a greater benefit of varenicline in those who use both alcohol and cigarettes, compared to those who just use alcohol.

This 16-week study was a phase two, randomized, double-blind, placebo-controlled trial comparing the effects of varenicline and medical management to medical management plus placebo for treatment of AUD. The 131 participants recruited (including 39 women) met DSM-IV-TR criteria for alcohol dependence and smoked at least 2 days a week. The intervention group was given varenicline titrated up to 1 mg twice a day, and both groups were seen for 12 medical management sessions for AUD, which is a behavioral intervention used by medical professionals to support medication adherence (4 sessions) and use strategies for achieving drinking goals (8 sessions).

The primary outcomes were reduction in drinking by percentage of heavy drinking days (PHDD) and no heavy drinking days (NHDD), defined as ≥ 5 standard drinks a day for men or ≥ 4 for women. One standard drink equaled a 12-ounce beer with an alcohol content of 5%, 5 ounces of wine (12% alcohol), or 1.5 ounces of distilled spirits (40% alcohol). Secondary outcomes were prolonged abstinence (28 days) from smoking, confirmed by plasma cotinine levels < 6 ng/mL.

RESULTS

The results of the primary outcome, PHDD, showed no significant difference in the overall sample between those on varenicline or placebo. However, there was a significant difference between the response of men and women in the study. PHDD in men showed a greater (but still non-significant) reduction than women, and the NHDD in men was nearly significant—29% on varenicline had NHDD vs 6% for placebo (95% CI, 0.22–1.03). Smoking outcomes showed a significant difference in prolonged abstinence from smoking for those on varenicline—13% vs 0% (p = 0.003). The only significantly different side effect was more abnormal dreaming in the varenicline group (43.8% vs 22.4%), which was experienced more often by women than men—women taking varenicline were 35% more likely than men to report this complaint.

Three adverse events happened in the varenicline group: an admission to alcohol rehabilitation, a hospitalization for suicidal ideation, and another hospitalization for blood pressure monitoring. Two adverse events happened with placebo: psychiatric hospitalization in one, and hospitalization for an infection in another. Women on varenicline were more likely to report abnormal dreams and to reduce or discontinue the medication than either men or women on placebo.

THE CARLAT TAKE

While the results are not robust, they point to a greater benefit in men with AUD than in women. However, the small number of women in the study limits this conclusion, and it could be that women don't tolerate treatment doses of varenicline as well.

PRACTICE IMPLICATIONS

More research is needed to investigate these gender differences in varenicline efficacy and tolerance. There isn't enough evidence to support varenicline's use as a treatment of AUD. Another take-home point is that, even without any other smoking cessation interventions, varenicline helped some people achieve prolonged abstinence from smoking.

PHARMACOTHERAPY DEVELOPMENTS

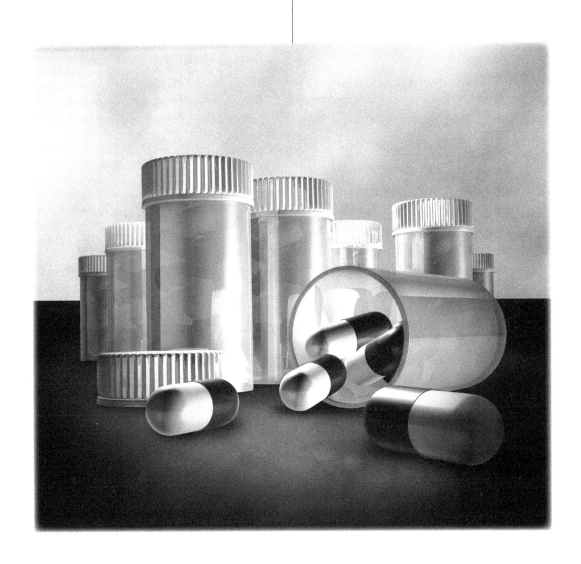

Olanzapine for Anorexia Nervosa

REVIEW OF: **Attia E, Steinglass JE, Walsh BT, et al. Olanzapine versus placebo in adult outpatients with anorexia nervosa: A randomized clinical trial. *Am J Psychiatry*. 2019 Jun 1;176(6):449–456.**

STUDY TYPE: **Randomized, double-blind, placebo-controlled trial**

ANTIPSYCHOTICS HAVE BEEN tried in anorexia since 1960, but their success has been mixed and often outweighed by their risks. Seven controlled trials have tested atypical antipsychotics in anorexia, and although most were positive, their pooled benefits were too small to be detected in a meta-analysis (Dodd M et al, *Psychother Psychosom* 2015;84(2):110–116). That leaves us with an uncertainty that is best answered by a larger controlled trial, which is where this new research comes in.

In this randomized placebo-controlled trial, researchers studied the effects of olanzapine on change in body weight and obsessionality in adult outpatients (n = 152) with anorexia nervosa for 16 weeks. Nearly all patients were female (96%) and most were taking psychotropics (41%, mainly antidepressants). Average BMI was 17 and Yale-Brown Obsessive Compulsive Scale (YBOCS) score was 16.5 (moderate severity). Olanzapine was started at 2.5 mg/day × 2 weeks, titrated to 5 mg/day × 2 weeks, and then increased to 10 mg/day as tolerated (average final dose 7.8 mg/day). Primary outcome measures were rate of change in body weight and rate of change in obsessionality measured by the YBOCS.

RESULTS

Relative to placebo, the olanzapine group experienced a significant increase of 0.165 BMI points, which is approximately 1 pound per month over the 16 weeks. Relative to placebo, the olanzapine group did not see a benefit in obsessionality or cognitive symptoms of anorexia and had significantly more concerns about body weight. Lab abnormalities and hospitalization rates did not differ between the groups.

THE CARLAT TAKE

This study's strengths include the large sample size and enrollment of diverse patients with various comorbidities that are more reflective of outpatient practice. The sample size is almost as large as all the past atypical antipsychotic studies of anorexia combined. The study's main weaknesses include the large dropout rate (45%) and a duration that was probably not long enough to detect lab abnormality differences. On the other hand, the dropout rate was similar for olanzapine and placebo, and the data were analyzed on an intent-to-treat basis.

PRACTICE IMPLICATIONS

Despite a positive result, these modest gains in weight do not inspire a ringing endorsement of olanzapine for anorexia. At least seven other controlled trials of olanzapine in anorexia have been published, and a meta-analysis of them did not find a hair of difference with olanzapine or with other antipsychotics (Cassioli E et al, *J Psychopharmacol* 2020;34(8):864–873). Reserve olanzapine for severe, treatment-resistant patients where weight restoration is essential, or for patients with anorexia who have comorbidities—like mood disorders—where olanzapine is indicated.

Another Black Eye for Prazosin in PTSD?

REVIEW OF: McCall WV, Pillai A, Case D, et al. A pilot, randomized clinical trial of bedtime doses of prazosin versus placebo in suicidal posttraumatic stress disorder patients with nightmares. *J Clin Psychopharmacol.* 2018 Dec;38(6):618–621.

STUDY TYPE: Randomized, double-blind, placebo-controlled trial

PRAZOSIN HAS BECOME a mainstay in the pharmacologic treatment of PTSD. A selective antagonist of the noradrenergic alpha-1 receptor, it has modest benefits in sleep and nightmares that are supported by around half a dozen clinical trials. That mainstay of practice was recently rocked by a large trial of twice-daily prazosin in (mainly male) military veterans that found no benefit for distressing dreams or sleep quality (Raskind M et al, *NEJM* 2018;378(6):507–517). But the study had flaws, particularly in the way that patients were selected to participate. Now we have a second report questioning prazosin's utility in PTSD.

The authors hypothesized that prazosin might reduce suicidality in patients with PTSD, based on prior research suggesting a link between insomnia and suicide. They randomized 20 civilians (17 women, 3 men) with PTSD to prazosin or placebo for 8 weeks. Prazosin was given at night in escalating doses as tolerated (the mean final dose was 5.5±3.5 mg qhs). Prior to randomization, the subjects were stabilized for at least 4 weeks on an SSRI or, if suffering from bipolar depression, at least 4 weeks on an FDA-approved bipolar medication. The primary outcome was suicidality, as measured by the Scale for Suicide Ideation (SSI) and the Columbia-Suicide Severity Rating Scale (C-SSRS). Secondary measures included the Disturbing Dreams and Nightmare Severity Index (DDNSI), the Insomnia Severity Index (ISI), and PTSD as measured by the PTSD-checklist-specific version.

RESULTS

The results were surprising. Contrary to expectations, the placebo group showed greater improvement on all measures, including nightmares and insomnia, but also on measures of depression and PTSD overall. However, the study had significant weaknesses that make it difficult to conclude much from these results. The sample size was small, and only 6 of the 20 subjects completed the full 8 weeks. The placebo response was also very high. Suicidality remitted *completely* on placebo, as measured by the SSI, but on prazosin it only declined 70%.

THE CARLAT TAKE

The placebo response has risen in the last 20 years, and that means we're seeing more studies like this where an otherwise effective treatment fails to separate from placebo. Transcranial magnetic stimulation, behavioral interventions for PTSD, and now prazosin have all shared this fate.

PRACTICE IMPLICATIONS

The lesson is to beware of media headlines that proclaim a common therapy ineffective. Sometimes the treatment is flawed; sometimes it's the study. In this case, we're not convinced that it's time to give up on prazosin in PTSD. After this study was released, a meta-analysis of six randomized controlled trials of prazosin in PTSD concluded that it treated PTSD with a small effect size for core PTSD symptoms, a medium effect on sleep, and a large effect on nightmares (Reist C et al, *CNS Spectr* 2020;25(1):1–7).

Is Ketamine Just Another Opiate?

REVIEW OF: **Williams NR, Heifets BD, Blasey C, et al. Attenuation of antidepressant effects of ketamine by opioid receptor antagonism.** *Am J Psychiatry*. **2018 Dec 1;175(12):1205–1215.**

STUDY TYPE: **Randomized, double-blind, placebo-controlled, crossover study**

KETAMINE'S RAPID ANTIDEPRESSANT effects have now been demonstrated in over two dozen double-blind, placebo-controlled trials, but how it works is less clear. For many years, NMDA receptor antagonism was thought responsible, but other NMDA antagonists have not worked well in depression. Another possibility is the endogenous opioid system, which is responsible for ketamine's analgesic effects. If that system is also involved in ketamine's antidepressant effects, then the opioid antagonist naltrexone ought to interfere with those benefits. This study sought to determine whether naltrexone would in fact dampen ketamine's benefits in depression.

Thirty subjects with chronic, highly refractory depression were enrolled (with a mean of 9.8 unsuccessful antidepressant trials). Each participant received, in random order, two separate IV infusions of ketamine 0.5 mg/kg—one preceded by naltrexone 50 mg and the other preceded by placebo. The primary outcome was reduction in depressive symptoms at post-infusion day 1. The dissociative effects of ketamine were examined as well.

RESULTS

When ketamine was given with a placebo, the response (58%) and remission (42%) rates for depression were high, but coadministration with naltrexone brought those rates to zero. In contrast, naltrexone did not have any discernible impact on ketamine's dissociative effects. Data collected on blinding suggested that participants were unable to discern when they were receiving naltrexone vs placebo.

The results were dramatic enough that the study was halted midway through for ethical reasons, so only 12 of the 30 subjects completed both arms.

THE CARLAT TAKE

Could ketamine be nothing more than an opiate masquerading as an NMDA receptor antagonist? While the opioid system appears critical to ketamine's antidepressant effects, that doesn't mean ketamine directly affects opioid receptors in the way that morphine or codeine does. Endogenous opioids have well-known mood elevating properties, and exercise and even placebo stimulate endogenous opioids.

However, the possibility of an opioid-like effect raises uncomfortable questions about potential withdrawal symptoms after stopping ketamine, or its branded cousin esketamine (Spravato). Furthering that concern is the fact that there were 3 suicides in the treatment arm after long-term esketamine was stopped in the registration trials. The suicides were not statistically significant, so they did not stop Spravato from getting FDA approval for treatment-resistant depression, but they raise red flags that have yet to be answered in light of this opioid finding.

PRACTICE IMPLICATIONS

While ketamine and its branded cousin esketamine (Spravato) treat depression, they do nothing to prevent it, so patients are increasingly placed on these medications long term. The data above suggest that some of these patients may be vulnerable to withdrawal problems, including worsening depression and suicidality, if ketamine or esketamine are ever stopped. Until that possibility is refuted, watch those patients closely.

Serotonin Syndrome Risks With Co-Prescription of Triptan Drugs and SSRIs or SNRIs

REVIEW OF: Orlova Y, Rizzoli P, Loder E. Association of coprescription of triptan antimigraine drugs and selective serotonin reuptake inhibitor or selective norepinephrine reuptake inhibitor antidepressants with serotonin syndrome. *JAMA Neurol.* 2018 May 1;75(5):566–572.

STUDY TYPE: Retrospective cohort study

IN 2006, THE FDA issued a warning that patients using either selective serotonin reuptake inhibitors or serotonin-norepinephrine reuptake inhibitors (SSRIs or SNRIs) together with triptan antimigraine drugs might be at a heightened risk for serotonin syndrome. Their advisory was based on 27 case reports of suspected serotonin syndrome in people who were prescribed a triptan along with one of these serotonergic antidepressants.

Because migraines are a common comorbidity in depressive and anxiety disorders, many of our patients are co-prescribed these medications. But what is the true risk for serotonin syndrome for these patients?

Orlova at the University of Florida and colleagues from Boston's Brigham and Women's Hospital completed a population-based study to evaluate this risk. They used electronic health records from over 6 million members in the Partners Research Data Registry to identify a cohort of 19,017 patients, who were prescribed both triptans and an SSRI or SNRI between 2001 and 2017, a total of 30,928 person-years of exposure.

RESULTS

Serotonin syndrome was suspected in 17 patients, and concurrent use of triptans and an SSRI/SNRI was confirmed in 7 of these. Serotonin syndrome was considered definite in 2 of those cases and possible in the other 5, yielding an incidence rate of 0.6–2.3 cases per 10,000 person-years of exposure.

The rate of co-prescription did not change after the 2006 FDA warning. Between 2001 and 2014, 21%–29% of triptan users were also prescribed an SSRI or SNRI.

THE CARLAT TAKE

Serotonin syndrome is hypothesized to involve activation of only serotonin 2A and 1A receptors. Triptans are primarily agonists for serotonin 1B and 1D receptors and do not activate serotonin 2A or 1A receptors. Thus, we doubt that triptans would increase the risk of serotonin syndrome.

PRACTICE IMPLICATIONS

The risk of serotonin syndrome with concomitant use of triptans and SSRIs or SNRIs appears to be very low. These results cast serious doubt on the validity of the 2006 FDA advisory and suggest that it should be reconsidered.

QTc Prolongation Risk Management in Hospital Patients

REVIEW OF: Vandael E, Vandenberk B, Willems R, et al. Risk management of hospitalized psychiatric patients taking multiple QTc-prolonging drugs. *J Clin Psychopharmacol.* 2017 Oct;37(5):540–545.

STUDY TYPE: **Prospective cohort study**

MANY OF THE medications we prescribe, most notably antipsychotics and antidepressants, have some risk of QTc prolongation. Since it's rare to have complications of a prolonged QTc interval—such as torsades de pointes and sudden cardiac death—clinics and hospitals typically don't screen for QTc prolongation using electrocardiograms (ECG).

This study evaluated the impact of combining two medications that are known to cause QTc prolongation, and attempted to stratify patients based on a baseline risk score calculation. The study population consisted of 152 patients in six psychiatric hospitals who were already taking 1 or more QTc-prolonging medications. All patients received a baseline ECG to see whether their existing medication was causing QTc prolongation. When a second torsadogenic medication was added, patients were given another ECG within 14 days. The most common medications prescribed in the study were mirtazapine, quetiapine, escitalopram, and trazodone.

RESULTS

How did adding these medications affect ECGs? Across all patients, there was a statistically significant increase (p = 0.032) in mean QTc interval from a norm of 409.1 ms to 411.8 ms with a single QTc-prolonging medication. At follow-up ECG, after the addition of a second QTc-prolonging medication, only 3 participants (2%) developed a prolonged QTc (≥ 450 ms for men and ≥ 470 ms for women). Only 8 patients (6.6%) had an increase in their QTc ≥ 30 ms, and no one had an increase in QTc ≥ 60 ms. No study participants experienced torsades de pointes or sudden cardiac death.

The study also explored potential predictors of QTc prolongation by assigning a risk score at baseline. This score, called the "RISQ-PATH score," was computed using the patient's age, sex, cardiac risk factors, and number of QTc-prolonging medications currently prescribed.

According to the RISQ-PATH score, 58 patients (38.2%) were considered high risk at baseline, and these patients had a significantly higher QTc interval in the follow-up ECG compared to low-risk patients (420.7 ms vs 406.2 ms, p < 0.001).

THE CARLAT TAKE

There is a direct correlation between the number of QTc-prolonging medications and a longer QTc interval. However, for most patients in this study, the absolute increase in QTc interval was very small, with only 2% of patients developing a prolonged QTc. And, regardless of the QTc prolongations, none of these patients developed any clinical symptoms attributable to the ECG changes. A risk score, such as the RISQ-PATH score, would be helpful in choosing which patients need ECG monitoring, but this test needs further validation before being used in the general psychiatric population. Also, since the problem may be greater among the elderly, these data may not be reassuring for a geropsychiatrist.

PRACTICE IMPLICATIONS

Combining QTc-prolonging medications can have an additive effect on the QTc interval, but the magnitude of this effect is small, with a very low probability of clinical consequences in most patients. While prudence would dictate avoiding such combinations, if the patient's symptoms require these medications, go ahead and prescribe them while monitoring the ECG. Exercise caution in patients with additional risks for QT interval prolongation, including those with congenital long QT syndrome, electrolyte abnormalities, or the elderly.

Varenicline and Bupropion: Soaring Again With EAGLES?

REVIEW OF: Anthenelli RM, Benowitz NL, West R, et al. Neuropsychiatric safety and efficacy of varenicline, bupropion, and nicotine patch in smokers with and without psychiatric disorders (EAGLES): A double-blind, randomised, placebo-controlled clinical trial. *Lancet*. 2016 Jun 18;387(10037):2507–2520.

STUDY TYPE: Randomized, double-blind, placebo-controlled trial

VARENICLINE (CHANTIX) AND bupropion (Zyban and others) are effective treatments for tobacco use disorder, but their use (and sales) took a big hit in 2009 when the FDA slapped both with black box warnings linking them to psychiatric complications, including suicidal ideation. Although these concerns did not appear in clinical trials, the FDA responded primarily to numerous post-marketing case reports. Clinicians began to steer clear of these agents, especially after a cottage industry cropped up suing for psychiatric damages purportedly caused by them. To allow removal of the warning, the FDA required the manufacturers of Chantix and Zyban (Pfizer and GlaxoSmithKline, respectively) to perform a sufficiently large randomized trial that adequately assessed these safety issues. The result is the massive and complicated Pfizer- and GSK-sponsored "EAGLES" trial—a somewhat tortured acronym of "Evaluating Adverse Events in a Global Smoking Cessation Study."

This randomized, double-blind clinical trial recruited 8,144 smokers ages 18–75 from 140 centers in 16 countries. Subjects were split into two cohorts, one with and the other without psychiatric disorders. Each cohort was then divided into four treatment groups in a 1:1:1:1 ratio: varenicline (target dose 1 mg BID), bupropion SR (150 mg BID), transdermal nicotine patch (21 mg/day with taper), or placebo. The treatment phase lasted 12 weeks, followed by a 12-week non-treatment follow-up phase. Subjects were assessed for both tobacco abstinence and for 16 categories of neuropsychiatric symptoms. The main goal was to determine whether the treatments differed in terms of serious psychiatric side effects.

RESULTS

Not surprisingly, there were more reported neuropsychiatric adverse events in the psychiatric cohort (5.8%) than in the non-psychiatric cohort (2.1%). However, the overall incidence of these events was the same in each of the four treatment groups. In fact, anxiety and depression symptoms improved about equivalently in all groups. The most common adverse events by treatment group were nausea (varenicline 25%), insomnia (bupropion 12%), abnormal dreams (nicotine patch 12%), and headache (placebo 10%). Rates of suicidal ideation and behavior overall were quite low, but in the psychiatric cohort they were non-significantly higher in the placebo and varenicline groups. The lone completed suicide was in the non-psychiatric placebo group.

All three of the active treatments were more effective for tobacco abstinence than placebo, but varenicline was superior to both bupropion and nicotine patch.

THE CARLAT TAKE

The EAGLES study described here has been criticized for its use of an unvalidated scale for adverse events. Further, the FDA raised concerns over inconsistencies in EAGLES' data collection, but ultimately found that, even when unreliable data were excluded, the results seemed consistent with the study's conclusions. As a result, the FDA removed the black box warning for varenicline, and it modified the warning for Zyban by removing language about serious psychiatric effects in patients quitting smoking.

PRACTICE IMPLICATIONS

These agents, particularly varenicline, can help patients stop smoking, and serious psychiatric adverse effects seem relatively rare. So, we can all breathe somewhat easier in prescribing varenicline and bupropion for smoking cessation. But as with all psychotropic agents, it would be prudent to employ reasonable screening, discussion of risks, and monitoring effects of these agents, particularly in patients who have preexisting psychiatric symptoms.

Does Augmenting Varenicline With Bupropion Work Better Than Varenicline Alone?

REVIEW OF: **Cinciripini PM, Minnix JA, Green CE, et al. An RCT with the combination of varenicline and bupropion for smoking cessation: Clinical implications for front line use.** *Addiction* **2018 Sep;113(9):1673–1682.**

STUDY TYPE: **Randomized, double-blind, placebo-controlled trial**

WE HAVE A good array of smoking cessation treatments to choose from, including nicotine replacement therapy (NRT), bupropion, and varenicline. Varenicline is the most effective monotherapy agent, somewhat better than bupropion and single-product NRT, and comparable to combination NRT. Theoretically, adding bupropion to varenicline would be even more effective. A couple of studies have tested this strategy with mixed results. This latest study attempted to further clarify the efficacy of this combination.

Researchers randomly assigned smokers (at least 1 pack per day) to three treatment arms: varenicline alone (n = 166), varenicline plus bupropion (n = 163), and placebo (n = 56). All participants were also given behavioral therapy (13 in-person individual 15-minute visits for smoking cessation counseling and 2 brief supportive telephone sessions) for 12 weeks of active treatment. They were then followed for 12 months. The primary outcome measure was abstinence at 1 year, which was verified by measuring expired carbon monoxide. The majority of participants were male (58%), and the average age was 49.

RESULTS

After 12 months, the quit rates were similar in the two active treatment groups. Beginning with the last 4 weeks of treatment, participants on varenicline alone had a continuous abstinence rate of 22.29% vs 20.25% for the varenicline + bupropion group. Both of these were superior to placebo, which had a continuous abstinence rate of 5.36%.

As expected, the rate of adverse events was higher in the varenicline + bupropion (98.1%) and varenicline-only (95.78%) groups compared with placebo (89.29%; p < 0.021). Specifically, varenicline + bupropion participants experienced decreased appetite, altered taste, and increased dry mouth, insomnia, creatinine, and edema compared with placebo. Varenicline-only participants had increased rates of abnormal dreams, diarrhea, and nausea compared with placebo.

THE CARLAT TAKE

While it's tempting to combine two effective treatments, it appears that adding bupropion to varenicline is no better than varenicline alone. Varenicline comes with a host of side effects, but if tolerated can help many people quit smoking.

PRACTICE IMPLICATIONS

While all smoking cessation agents can be used as first-line treatment, in Carlat's *Medication Fact Book for Psychiatric Practice,* we lay out an approach that starts with nicotine replacement therapy, and then moves on to either varenicline or bupropion. These results are in line with that approach.

Can Buprenorphine Improve
PTSD Symptoms?

REVIEW OF: Lake EP, Mitchell BG, Shorter DI, et al. Buprenorphine for the treatment of posttraumatic stress disorder. *Am J Addict.* 2019 Feb;28(2):86–91.

STUDY TYPE: **Retrospective case series**

FOR MANY YEARS, the mainstay of treatment for PTSD has been the SSRI class of medications, but many of our patients still suffer crippling symptoms despite optimal antidepressant medication dosing. PTSD is often accompanied by opioid misuse, sometimes in an effort to self-treat the hyperarousal and hypervigilance related to PTSD. So, can treatments like buprenorphine/naloxone that target opioid receptors also have an effect on PTSD symptoms?

This retrospective study looked at three groups of patients with PTSD treated at VA medical centers over a 6-year period—those receiving SSRIs, buprenorphine/naloxone, and full-agonist opioids. Patients could only have been receiving 1 of these medications during the study period. A total of 2,015 patients were identified, out of which 55 patients were selected for each group after applying the inclusion criteria and then using a random number generator. The subjects were mostly white (76.4%) and male (88.5%), with an average age of 43. PTSD symptoms were assessed using either the PTSD Checklist for Clinicians (PCL-C) or the VA Primary Care PTSD Screen (PC-PTSD)—the PCL-C scores were converted to the PC-PTSD scale for the analysis. This new standardized score was a 4-point scale, with 1 being minimal and 4 being maximal symptoms. A score of 3 or 4 is considered a "positive" screening for PTSD. The primary outcome was the most recent standardized PTSD rating scale score, with a secondary outcome of change in score from initial to most recent assessment.

RESULTS

The buprenorphine group had the best final standardized PTSD score, significantly better than the SSRI group (2.473 vs 3.164; p = 0.048). There was no significant difference between the final scores of the SSRI vs full-agonist opioid groups or between the buprenorphine vs full-agonist opioid groups. For the change from initial to final standardized PTSD score, the buprenorphine group also did the best, with significantly greater change in scores compared to the SSRI group (p = 0.026), and again no differences were found in the other two group comparisons.

THE CARLAT TAKE

The results are interesting but should be taken with a grain of salt. This study was set up as a retrospective chart review, not a prospective efficacy study. The time intervals for rating scale assessments weren't standardized, there was no standard length of treatment, and the study did not control for confounding factors such as age, comorbid conditions, or concurrent psychotherapy.

PRACTICE IMPLICATIONS

At most, this study gives us more confidence in using buprenorphine/naloxone when treating comorbid PTSD and opioid use disorder, but randomized controlled trials are needed to establish efficacy in PTSD treatment.

PSYCHOTHERAPY INTERVENTIONS

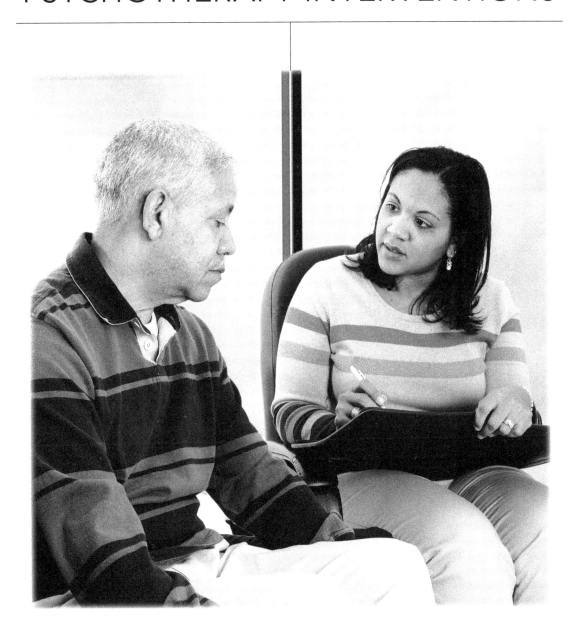

Are All Psychotherapies for Anorexia Created Equal?

REVIEW OF: Zeeck A, Herpertz-Dahlmann B, Friederich HC, et al. Psychotherapeutic treatment for anorexia nervosa: A systematic review and network meta-analysis. *Front Psychiatry*. 2018 May 1;9:158.

STUDY TYPE: Meta-analysis of randomized controlled trials

PSYCHOTHERAPY IS THE main treatment for anorexia nervosa, but which type works best? Several therapies have good evidence in this population, but they differ in their models and methods, and head-to-head comparisons among them are rare. To overcome that limitation, this study used a technique called "network meta-analysis," which evaluates different treatments based on how they measured up against a common comparison group. For example, suppose that cognitive behavioral therapy (CBT) and family therapy have never been directly compared to each other but both have been compared to supportive therapy. A network meta-analysis would compare CBT to family therapy based on how each fared relative to supportive therapy.

Only a handful of therapies have good evidence to work in anorexia, and most of them were included in this study. Effective therapies had two common ingredients: a focus on weight restoration and work on psychosocial factors. It was in the psychosocial focus that the therapies differed, which ranged from skill building (CBT), relationship dynamics (focal psychodynamic therapy, interpersonal psychotherapy), family work, and supportive psychotherapy (specialist supportive clinical management). The family therapies empowered parents to re-feed their child, and then progressed to work on family dynamics (systemic family therapy) or adolescent development (family-based treatment and the Maudsley model) as normal weight was restored.

RESULTS

No single therapy was more effective than the others in this analysis of 18 randomized controlled trials. The authors followed that up with another new-fangled technique, called "standardized mean change analysis," which compared the degree of weight gain among all of the therapies after 1 year of treatment. This analysis allowed naturalistic studies to be included, bringing the total number of trials to 38. Again, no single therapy stood out, but weight gain was more rapid with inpatient vs outpatient treatment, and overall weight gain was greater in adolescent studies than it was for adults (inpatient: 1.4 pounds/week for adolescents, 1.2 pounds/week for adults; outpatient: 0.42 pounds/week for adolescents, 0.23 pounds/week for adults).

THE CARLAT TAKE

The authors suggested that some therapies may be superior for certain subgroups of anorexia. Most successful therapies for adolescents involved the family, while individual therapy was the mainstay for adults with anorexia. Adolescents with significant obsessive-compulsive symptoms had greater benefit with systemic family therapy than family-based treatment. For severe anorexia, the Maudsley model was more effective than specialist supportive clinical management.

PRACTICE IMPLICATIONS

While the outcomes for these therapies were similar, this does not mean that any psychotherapy will work for anorexia. These are highly structured therapies with specific behavioral and psychological techniques. When making referrals, psychiatrists should look for therapists that use evidence-based methods, and adolescents may do better with a family approach. Once in therapy, weight gain of 0.23–1.4 pounds/week can be considered a successful outcome.

Mindfulness Therapy for Adult ADHD

REVIEW OF: Janssen L, Kan CC, Carpentier PJ, et al. **Mindfulness-based cognitive therapy v. treatment as usual in adults with ADHD: A multicentre, single-blind, randomised controlled trial.** *Psychol Med.* 2019 Jan;49(1):55–65.

STUDY TYPE: Randomized, single-blind, active-controlled trial

MEDICATIONS ARE THE first-line treatment for adult ADHD, and the efficacy of psychosocial therapies is less well defined. Mindfulness-based therapy showed promise for adult ADHD in a recent meta-analysis, but there were flaws and significant differences between the included studies (Janssen L et al, *BMC Psychiatry* 2015;15:216).

The current study was a single-blind, randomized controlled trial of mindfulness-based cognitive behavioral therapy (MBCT) as an adjunct to treatment as usual (TAU) in 120 patients with adult ADHD. Both groups received TAU, which consisted of various combinations of medication, psychoeducation, and skills training. The intervention group received 8 weekly sessions of MBCT and a 6-hour silent day of mindfulness. Each MBCT session was 2.5 hours long and consisted of meditation exercises, cognitive behavioral techniques, psychoeducation, and group discussions. For the silent day, study subjects spent 6 hours completing various meditation activities, eating lunch, and having a tea break. Mindfulness practice was encouraged outside of the sessions for 30 minutes a day.

RESULTS

Patients in the MBCT group had significant reductions in clinician-rated and self-reported ADHD symptoms that persisted for 6 months. Significantly more patients in the MBCT group (27%) experienced a ≥ 30% reduction in symptoms compared with the TAU group (5%) (p = 0.001). The two groups were similar in their utilization of TAU, although those in the mindfulness group were less likely to make changes to their medications.

THE CARLAT TAKE

Although the results are encouraging, the study had several limitations. Participants were not blinded to the treatment, so placebo effects cannot be completely ruled out. No data were collected on patients who were excluded or declined to participate in the study, raising the possibility that the sample was enriched and limiting the generalizability of the results.

PRACTICE IMPLICATIONS

This study raises the quality of evidence in support of mindfulness therapy in adult ADHD. Mindfulness is reasonable to recommend as an adjunct to medication, and as a solo treatment for patients who cannot tolerate or do not respond to medication.

A CBT App for Refractory Depression

REVIEW OF: **Mantani A, Kato T, Furukawa TA, et al. Smartphone cognitive behavioral therapy as an adjunct to pharmacotherapy for refractory depression: Randomized controlled trial.** *J Med Internet Res.* **2017 Nov 3;19(11):e373.**

STUDY TYPE: **Randomized, single-blind, parallel-group trial**

MOBILE PHONES HAVE allowed the introduction of guided, self-help cognitive behavioral therapy (CBT) for depression with enhanced accessibility, efficiency, and affordability. Several meta-analyses suggest that computers can augment face-to-face psychotherapy and even work on their own through self-guided programs. Most of those studies involved patients with mild to moderate depression, which leaves open the question of how well this approach would work in more severe cases.

This study tested a self-guided mobile app in patients with moderate to severe depression who had not responded to at least 1 antidepressant trial. The Japanese app, called Kokoro, used cartoon characters to present concepts from CBT, including self-monitoring, behavioral activation, and cognitive restructuring.

The authors randomized 164 patients to an intervention group (medication switch plus Kokoro app) and control group (medication switch only). Although the treatments were not blinded, the outcomes were assessed with blinded raters.

RESULTS

After 9 weeks, the intervention group showed greater improvement in the Patient Health Questionnaire-9, the primary outcome measure (p < 0.001). Rates of remission (18% vs 10%) and response (32% vs 18%) were also greater, and the magnitude of the benefit compared favorably with the effect sizes seen in antidepressant trials.

In the second phase of the study, both groups were given access to the app for an additional 2 months. After that time, both groups had similar depression scores. The intervention group maintained their gains, and the control group caught up.

Most patients stayed engaged with the 8-session app, but that engagement was not entirely self-driven. Each week, participants received a brief, personalized email congratulating them on their progress.

THE CARLAT TAKE

This study demonstrates significant benefits for this CBT app in difficult-to-treat depression. Its strengths include a randomized controlled design, blinded ratings, and high levels of engagement and completion. The main limitation is the lack of blinding in the treatment arm, which makes it difficult to rule out a placebo effect. By making changes to medications in both groups at the start of the trial, the authors attempted to minimize expectancy effects.

PRACTICE IMPLICATIONS

For clinicians, the main limitation may be the inaccessibility of the Japanese-language app, a common problem in this type of research. Most of the available mental health apps are untested, and most of the tested apps are not available. A reasonable substitute is IntelliCare, a suite of CBT-based apps made free through NIMH funding (https://intellicare.cbits. northwestern.edu). In a recent randomized controlled trial, IntelliCare was compared to a waitlist control for treatment of anxiety and depression in primary care settings with significant positive results (Graham AK et al, *JAMA Psychiatry* 2020;e201011).

CBT vs Pharmacotherapy for Childhood Anxiety

REVIEW OF: Wang Z, Whiteside SPH, Sim L, et al. Comparative effectiveness and safety of cognitive behavioral therapy and pharmacotherapy for childhood anxiety disorders: A systematic review and meta-analysis. *JAMA Pediatr.* 2017 Nov 1;171(11):1049–1056.

STUDY TYPE: Systematic review and meta-analysis

MANAGING CHILDHOOD ANXIETY can sometimes leave clinicians in a quandary. There is a paucity of evidence comparing treatment approaches, and current guidelines on the subject are old and make inconsistent recommendations. To address this dilemma, researchers at the Mayo Clinic performed a systematic review and meta-analysis comparing pharmacotherapy with cognitive behavioral therapy (CBT) in children with anxiety disorders.

Investigators identified 115 studies with a total of 7,719 participants. All studies evaluated CBT, pharmacotherapy, or the combination of both for treatment of a diagnosed childhood anxiety disorder. The average participant age was 9.2 years (range 5.4 to 16.1), and slightly over half (55.6%) were female. Data were pooled using a random-effects meta-analysis.

RESULTS

Selective serotonin reuptake inhibitors (SSRIs) had significantly better outcomes than placebo for reduction in primary anxiety symptoms reported by parents or clinicians, as well as increased remission (relative risk [RR] 2.04) and response (RR 1.96). Likewise, when compared with placebo, serotonin-norepinephrine reuptake inhibitors (SNRIs) also had a significantly greater reduction in clinician-reported primary anxiety symptoms. The use of tricyclic antidepressants or benzodiazepines was not associated with a significant improvement in anxiety symptoms.

Treatment with CBT compared with no therapy significantly improved primary anxiety symptoms reported by clinicians, parents, and children, as well as remission (RR 4.08) and response (RR 4.72). Moreover, combining CBT with an SSRI resulted in significantly better response rates than treatment with an SSRI alone.

Mild or moderate adverse effects were reported with medication use but not with CBT. However, none of the trials were large enough or long enough to evaluate suicide risk with SSRIs or SNRIs.

THE CARLAT TAKE

This study provides insight into optimal treatment strategies for children with anxiety disorders. SSRIs or CBT are both effective therapies; SNRIs may also be useful alternatives to SSRIs, although the evidence supporting their efficacy is less robust. This study also supports the premise that there is an added benefit in combining CBT with pharmacotherapy. However, the authors caution that more research is needed to evaluate the comparative effectiveness of therapies—specifically, head-to-head evaluations of medication and CBT.

PRACTICE IMPLICATIONS

Importantly, these results allow clinicians to offer patients and their families several options for effective treatment of childhood anxiety. For most patients, we would suggest that offering a choice between pharmacotherapy or CBT is the best approach, explaining the risks and benefits of both. This allows patient and family preferences to guide the development of a treatment plan.

Exposure Therapy Efficacious for PTSD Co-Occurring With Alcohol Use Disorder

REVIEW OF: Norman SB, Trim R, Haller M, et al. Efficacy of integrated exposure therapy vs integrated coping skills therapy for comorbid posttraumatic stress disorder and alcohol use disorder: A randomized clinical trial. *JAMA Psychiatry*. 2019 Apr 24;76(8):791–799.

STUDY TYPE: Randomized, single-blind, active-controlled trial

P ATIENTS WITH CO-OCCURRING post-traumatic stress disorder (PTSD) and alcohol use disorder (AUD) have worse outcomes compared to patients with either diagnosis alone. Integrated approaches, in which both diagnoses are simultaneously addressed, are viewed as best practice. Providers, however, are often hesitant to offer prolonged exposure, an evidence-based therapy for PTSD, to dually diagnosed patients for fear that directly addressing patients' trauma might worsen their drinking. This study is the first randomized trial to compare two therapies targeting both disorders: integrated prolonged exposure (I-PE) vs integrated coping skills without exposure (I-CS).

In the study, 119 veterans were randomly assigned to 12–16 sessions of either I-PE or I-CS. Subjects were primarily male (n = 107), and the majority had experienced several trauma events—both related and not related to combat. Primary outcomes were assessed for both PTSD symptom severity and percentage of heavy drinking days (PHDD), which were measured via the Clinician-Administered PTSD Scale for DSM-5 (CAPS-5) and Timeline Followback questionnaires, respectively. Data were collected prior to treatment, post-treatment, and at 3 and 6 months following treatment.

RESULTS

Congruent with prior studies, PTSD severity decreased in both arms over time, and there was a significantly greater reduction in the I-PE group (p = 0.002). Regarding drinking outcomes, however, both arms were almost identical (p = 0.91). Encouragingly, regardless of whether the therapy involved exposure, PHDD dropped from approximately 50% to 20% by the end of the study, and there was a corresponding increase in days abstinent as well.

THE CARLAT TAKE

Prolonged exposure is one of the best treatments we have for PTSD, and this study helps show that it should not be withheld from patients with co-occurring AUD, especially when delivered in an integrated format that can also address alcohol use.

PRACTICE IMPLICATIONS

Our dual-diagnosis patients are often the most difficult to treat. Prolonged exposure therapy is an effective treatment for PTSD but can be very difficult for anyone to go through. This study confirms that prolonged exposure can be helpful for all patients, even those with active AUD.

New Hope: CBT for Internet and Computer Game Addiction

REVIEW OF: **Wölfling K, Müller KW, Dreier M, et al. Efficacy of short-term treatment of internet and computer game addiction: A randomized clinical trial. JAMA Psychiatry. 2019 Jul 10;76(10):1018–1025.**

STUDY TYPE: **Randomized, single-blind effectiveness trial**

WHILE MANY OF us likely spend far too much time on our various devices—whether for fun or for work—between 0.3% and 1% of the general population might qualify for an internet gaming disorder (Przybylski AK et al, *Am J Psychiatry* 2017;174(3):230–236). Defined as excessive preoccupation with online gaming despite negative life consequences, internet gaming disorder was identified in the 2013 publication of the DSM-5 as a condition warranting more clinical research and experience before it might be considered for inclusion as a formal disorder. In a recent multicenter randomized clinical trial, researchers evaluated the effectiveness of short-term cognitive behavioral therapy (CBT) for internet addiction.

The study randomly assigned 143 patients with DSM-5-proposed research criteria for internet and computer game disorder to short-term CBT (n = 72) or waitlist control (n = 71) and followed them for 6 months. The mean age was 26.2 years, and most participants were single, high school educated, and unemployed. All were male, which was intentionally reflective of the preponderance of treatment seekers.

The treatment group underwent 15 weekly groups of manualized CBT and up to 8 individual sessions that conceptualized their disorder as resulting from an interaction of individual factors, features of online activity, dysfunctional coping strategies, and disorder-specific cognitive biases. The primary outcome was remission based on a self-report measure, the Assessment of Internet and Computer Game Addiction (AICA-S). Secondary outcomes included time spent gaming or online, psychosocial functioning, and depressive symptoms.

RESULTS

The researchers found 69.4% of patients in short-term CBT achieved remission compared with 23.9% of those waitlisted (p < 0.001). There was a greater likelihood of remission in short-term CBT vs waitlist after controlling for age, baseline severity, and comorbidity (adjusted odds ratio 10.10; 95% CI 3.69–27.65). Both groups had improved depression ratings, which may have reflected repeat assessments and the prospect of future treatment for those waitlisted. At 6-month follow-up of half the patients in the short-term CBT group, 80.6% were in remission, but the authors claim this result is difficult to interpret owing to high rates of study dropout and the fact that follow-up data were not sought for the control group.

THE CARLAT TAKE

The results of this study offer hope for effective treatment of internet and computer game addiction. Still, more research is needed to better define these conditions, examine treatments among women, and compare short-term CBT with other treatments.

PRACTICE IMPLICATIONS

When managing a patient struggling with problematic gaming and/or internet use, consider CBT as a treatment option. This adds to the data that CBT is an effective treatment for a wide range of addictive disorders.

About Carlat Publishing

CARLAT PUBLISHING was founded by Daniel Carlat, MD. Its flagship publication is *The Carlat Psychiatry Report.* Dr. Carlat is an associate clinical professor of psychiatry at Tufts University. He is also the author of *Drug Metabolism in Psychiatry: A Clinical Guide, The Psychiatric Interview,* and *Unhinged,* and co-author of *The Medication Fact Book for Psychiatric Practice.*

For more information, visit www.thecarlatreport.com.

Contact us at:
info@thecarlatreport.com
866-348-9279

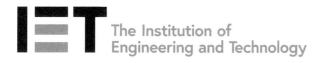
The Institution of
Engineering and Technology

Guide to
Smart Homes for
Electrical Installers

█ Publication information

Published by The Institution of Engineering and Technology, London, United Kingdom

The Institution of Engineering and Technology is registered as a Charity in England & Wales (no. 211014) and Scotland (no. SCO38698).

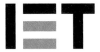

The Institution of Engineering and Technology is the institution formed by the joining together of the IEE (The Institution of Electrical Engineers) and the IIF (The Institution of Incorporated Engineers).

© 2021 The Institution of Engineering and Technology

First published 2021 (978-1-78561-654-9)

Copies of this publication may be obtained from:
PO Box 96
Stevenage
SG1 2SD, UK
Tel: +44 (0)1438 767328
Email: sales@theiet.org
www.electrical.theiet.org/books

ISBN 978-1-78561-654-9 (paperback)
ISBN 978-1-78561-653-2 (electronic)

Typeset in the UK by the Institution of Engineering and Technology, Stevenage
Printed in the UK by Elanders Ltd, Merlin Way, New York Business Park,
Newcastle Upon Tyne, TW NE 27 0QG

⬛ Contents

Contents

Contents

▬ Acknowledgements

The Institution of Engineering and Technology (IET) acknowledges the contribution made by the following individuals and organizations in the development of this document:

Technical Author

Allan Burns (Telemental)

Technical Committee

Peter Boait (De Montfort University)

Simon Buddle CEng MIET (CEDIA EMEA)

Paul Chaffers MIET (NAPIT)

Dan Milne (Wiise)

Phil Williams (LCL Awards)

Certsure LLP

Electrical Contractor's Association (ECA)

Loxone

Scolmore International Ltd

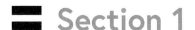 **Section 1**

Introduction

1.1 Scope

The definition of a smart home is complicated. For the purposes of this Guide, a smart home is a home that has a layer or layers of technology between the user and the systems within it. The different varieties of smart home will be illustrated throughout this Guide.

This Guide will help someone with electrical installation skills to identify and organize the elements that need to be incorporated when designing and specifying a smart home containing wired or wireless technology. It will support an electrical installer as they take on the extra duties, possibilities and liabilities entailed in smart home technology installation and support.

It cannot explain all the technology and processes that might be required, as these are application- and product-specific. Upskilling through training, and manufacturers' guidance, will be required continually, to keep up to date with developments.

This Guide is designed to help you understand what smart home technology is and give you confidence in specifying and installing it.

Smart measures span a whole spectrum of complexity. Wireless devices performing a single task will not require the same diligence as a fully featured, wired smart home. This Guide aims to prepare you for the latter and assumes that you will trim your efforts to fit more straightforward projects.

1.2 Who is this Guide for?

There is a rapidly growing opportunity for smart home installations in the UK. Smart homes offer householders a means to secure the latest technology; however, not all the devices are 'plug and play'. Many require input from competent electrical installers. That input could be as simple as running a new cable to a new point or installing a power socket with USB (universal serial bus) charging outlets, or it could be the design or reorganization of all the technology in the home. In this Guide, any actions taken that support or facilitate smart devices, or have smart outcomes, will be referred to as 'smart measures'. The term 'smart measure' includes smart devices.

It is likely that you, the electrical installer, will be the person called upon to install smart home technology. Perhaps a 'life moment trigger' will occur, such as a broken heating programmer. This is a great opportunity to do something 'smart' that is better for the electrical installer, the client and the environment.

There is huge variation in energy efficiency across British homes. The UK has a housebuilding programme and an important energy-saving agenda that also incentivises energy-saving retro-fit measures for our existing buildings. Live policies pushing for more energy-efficient homes include the Clean Growth Strategy, the Energy Performance of Buildings Directive and the minimum energy efficiency standards. Signposts to these can be found in Appendix C.

There are already lots of subsidy schemes operated by local authorities and we can expect to see more. These are likely to require people who have the skills to work with smart technology.

Existing trades with skills and experience that might be transferred into the smart home sector include:

(a) electrical installers; and
(b) fire and security alarm installers.

The scope of devices and applications being supported by or transformed into smart home technology is already large and is growing rapidly. Section 2.2 of this Guide illustrates these in detail.

This Guide is aimed at competent electrical installers who would like to take the opportunity to enter the smart home installation market. To be a trusted, informed voice in this area requires the practitioner to be knowledgeable and well-prepared. This Guide will walk you through the things you need to know: from your first contact with the home owner; to talking about their needs; through installation; and onto how to generate appropriate documents to support the installation.

This Guide assumes that the final implementation of any bespoke or fixed-wiring electrical system will be reviewed and carried out by a competent electrical installer. The standards for competency are discussed in the 18th Edition of the IET Wiring Regulations (BS 7671:2018+A1:2020) or the *Building standards technical handbook 2019: domestic* in Scotland. Signposts to further resources relating to smart home installation can be found in Appendix C.

1.3 What is different for the smart home installer?

1.3.1 More homework

Smart home technology offers solutions for the householder and opportunities for the installer, but can be more complex to specify and install. If you're carrying out a big project, you will need to carefully document your conversations with the householder, agree the specifications and manage expectations.

Installing smart measures will often mean going beyond the expectations of other trades and professions. There will be more explaining to do, right through the process from start to finish, to everyone involved in the process.

Becoming a smart home installer demands that you build upon the skills, knowledge and experience you developed as an electrical installer. The equipment you were familiar with for any given application might now have a connected element to it. That 'connectedness' might require specialist knowledge in such areas as IT and system integration. The electrical installation may also need consideration beyond protective earthing designed to protect people from electric shock, into functional earthing and bonding to minimize electromagnetic interference (EMI), for the purposes of optimizing performance. This Guide will summarize key elements and provide signposts to relevant standards (Appendix B) and further resources for knowledge and training (Appendix C).

Smart homes will offer more opportunities for ongoing relationships with the householder to help them manage and maintain their smart systems. In addition, it is still relatively early days for smart home technology, so products could become obsolete. You will therefore need a sincere and sustained interest to keep up with the technology.

1.3.2 More responsibility

Smart home products typically take repetitive control out of the householder's hands, so the installer of these products arguably becomes more responsible for consequences. Imagine a client presenting you with their electricity bill, which is four times higher than the year before you installed smart heating controls? Or perhaps a bill for a crushed car bonnet because the garage door mechanism was labelled incorrectly? There are many implications that mean you may need to review your trade insurance.

The situation is new for householders too. Larger jobs will need an extended handover or even a training session with householders. Additionally, being on call to answer any questions they have about their new systems may significantly change the way you allocate hours to, and charge for, jobs.

Section 1 – Introduction

Cyber security and the General Data Protection Regulation (GDPR) are also new areas that a smart electrical installer will need to consider. There are penalties for compromising a client's data security – and smart home systems may do that if they are not set up properly. Section 6.9.1 gives more guidance on how to approach this issue.

Smart electrical installers will be carrying out more work with home networks. A failed home network can be very problematic for the householder and the electrical installer who works on it will naturally find themself on the list of suspects if it goes wrong. You must therefore ask yourself if you know enough about smart installation to be able to deal with that situation.

1.3.3 Potentially, more revenue

Note the following:

(a) specialisms can command higher rates.
(b) smart electrical installers will have access to distribution streams with higher margins. Partnerships with high-end manufacturers can mean greater profit margins.
(c) smart electrical installers will have access to new markets. As more construction sectors are overhauled to incorporate smart measures, smaller contractors proficient with these technologies might gain a competitive edge over more established firms.
(d) smart homes and future-readying are increasingly in clients' minds: they will be attracted to practitioners who can deliver them.
(e) a new work stream for the support and maintenance of installed systems may develop.
(f) ask yourself the question: where will your business be if you don't take the opportunity, but your competitors do?

1.4 What is a smart home?

The first paragraph of this Guide offers a definition of a smart home – but a smart home installer should continue to ask the question. Is it simply having devices that can talk to one another, or make 'smart' decisions on behalf of a person? Or is it made up of systems that can be monitored and automated by the occupant through digital devices? We also now have the expectation that these devices should be connected to the internet and to each other – and this could become the feature that dominates the market.

Smart home projects can be:

(a) retrofit: a project where the smart measures are an addition to an existing installation. These can be wired or wireless, depending on circumstances and requirement.
(b) new build: a project where smart measures are designed in tandem with the environment being built. These tend to be wired, as the opportunity is open, but costs and requirement may still favour wireless technology.
(c) future build: a project that ignores all the old habits and conventions to do the best possible job with the available technology. This concept is still taking shape. It is characterized by co-dependency and the sharing of resources between buildings. A large number of such buildings would become a 'smart town' or 'smart city'.

1.5 Smart home benefits

Householders should rightly expect that living in a smart home packed with smart measures would bring advantages that improve their quality of life in some way.

There are two broad categories of smart measure:

1. smart home lifestyle products; and
2. smart home energy management products.

Note: Lifestyle can be a symptom of physical circumstances, such as a user's need for accessibility.

There is considerable overlap between the two categories. They can provide:

(a) more time, as some smart technology reduces day-to-day chores and inconveniences;

(b) personalization of the home: for example, through bespoke lighting;

(c) a potentially improved quality of life for vulnerable people, for example, the elderly, through assisted living technology;

(d) improvements in health: for example, air quality can be monitored and conditioned;

(e) benefits for wellness and productivity: for example, lighting colour temperature can be modulated to complement time of day and activity;

(f) increased economy: for example, metering and energy management can reduce bills;

(g) greater convenience: the ability to monitor and control the home remotely, particularly through security alarms and features;

(h) potential increase in home value;

(i) potential revenue from energy production in the home;

(j) potential savings for energy management in the home, giving access to time of use (TOU) tariffs and other tariff incentives;

(k) enhanced security; and

(l) a reduced impact on the environment, through the smarter use of utilities and the potential to co-ordinate the generation, storage and distribution of energy.

In addition to these general benefits, smart home benefits can be very specific to the individual. For example, an internet doorbell may be the ideal option for someone taking part in conference calls whilst expecting lots of deliveries. Smart plugs for switching appliances on and off are beneficial for those with back pain or other mobility issues.

1.6 Making a home future-ready

There is increasing awareness in the construction industry that buildings should be designed to allow the inclusion of new smart measures. Legislation such as the Energy Performance of Buildings Directive (EPBD – an EU initiative) is intended to commit volunteer member states to adopting building regulations that promote future-readiness. Signposts to this legislation and more can be found in Appendix C.

This Guide will show how to assess a client's ongoing needs. This creates a responsibility to identify and make contingency for new requirements that buildings might face in their lifetime, including questions of energy, materials and connectivity. These aspects are discussed in the Sections that follow.

1.6.1 Transport

Electric vehicle (EV) sales are growing fast and look set to keep increasing. The Office for Low Emission Vehicles (OLEV) has pledged to update Building Regulations to mandate that all new residential developments must contain enabling cabling for charge points in homes, in line with the recommendations in the EPBD. It is therefore likely that EV infrastructure, i.e. cables or ducts for cables, will become compulsory for new build homes. EVs can charge at currents that require a dedicated circuit.

Section 1 – Introduction

Getting an adequately sized cable or duct to the likely charge point location so that the client can install the best charge point available when they need it makes sense and works towards compliance with Approved Document Part L: *Conservation of fuel and power* of the Building Regulations.

1.6.2 Heating and cooling

Part L of the Building Regulations sets standards for the designers of new and existing buildings in terms of energy efficiency. While not responsible for the overall heat loss in the building, an informed electrical installer is able at least to lead with respect to the following requirements of Part L (L1A, 2.22):

> *In order to facilitate incorporation of improvements in system efficiencies and the integration with low and zero carbon technologies, the designer should:*
>
> *a. consider heating system designs that use low distribution temperatures; and*
> *b. where multiple systems serve the same end use,* ***organise the control strategies such that priority is given to the least carbon-intensive option****;*
> ***Note:*** *For example, where a solar hot water system is available,* ***use controls that make best use of the available solar energy****.*
> *c. consider* ***making the dwelling easily adaptable by facilitating the integration of additional low and zero carbon technologies at a later date****. Providing appropriate facilities at the construction stage can make subsequent enhancements much easier and cheaper, e.g. providing capped off connections that can link into a planned community heating scheme.*

In line with this, Appendix C of Lot 20 (a subdivision of items covered by the European Ecodesign Directive) phased out non-smart electric heaters. From 1st January 2018, all heaters must have:

(a) electronic time and temperature controls;
(b) open window sensing;
(c) predictive start; and
(d) remote control.

1.6.3 Communication

Home communication methods include:

(a) mobile phones – increasingly channelled through the router;
(b) skype/video-conferencing;
(c) device-to-device calling: for example, the Internet of Things (IoT);
(d) direct voice control: for example, the Amazon Alexa virtual assistant function; and
(e) landlines.

With respect to item (e), BT intends all its customers to be using fully digital telephone services by 2025. Voluntary migrations are scheduled from 2022, with a complete swap-over from the old analogue format planned for 2025. Secondary outlets wired in old six-core phone cables won't work after that, and an internet protocol (IP) phone will need to be connected to the internet connection.

We can also expect more traffic through the home broadband, particularly WiFi, and any designer should allow for that.

Figure 1.1   The shape of modern home communication

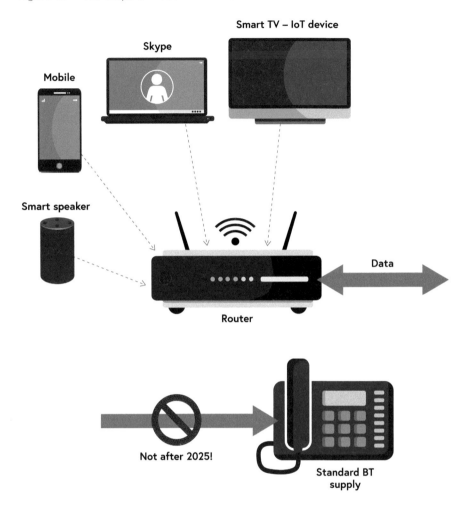

1.6.4   Entertainment

Home entertainment includes:

(a) artificial intelligence (AI) functions, such as Alexa or Google Home;
(b) online and multimedia gaming;
(c) streamed music and TV; and
(d) dedicated media sets: for example, Sky Q.

All these will require infrastructure to support them, and reasonable WiFi as a minimum. Very likely, wired internet will be needed to increase performance.

In addition, virtual and augmented reality devices are becoming better and more affordable. Where might your client want to use these when they become mainstream for entertainment? What infrastructure will these require?

1.6.5   Energy efficiency and energy management

Householders have always wanted to save money on bills. The last two decades have seen a tremendous upturn in the adoption of technological measures to assist with this, with the most prolific measure being solar photovoltaics (PV).

Section 1 – Introduction

The domestic PV application has developed to include auxiliary products such as energy capture for hot water, in which excess generated energy is diverted through an immersion heater so that it cannot escape to the grid.

PV has always been limited by the fact that the sun does not shine all the time. However, electrical energy storage (EES) technology is now able to spread the energy out over the dark spells too.

Figure 1.2   Solar peak versus morning and evening demand for electric energy

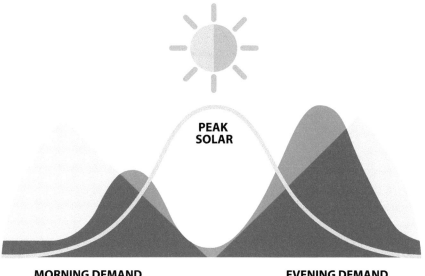

The National Grid is undergoing transformation to accommodate and take advantage of these changes. The exact form this will take is uncertain, but we can assume that domestic householders will have the opportunity to join in. Householders will be able to choose from tariffs that will reward them for having microgeneration (PV, wind or hydro) and storage on-site. TOU tariffs, which can vary rates according to times, will reward participants who co-ordinate their use and generation with wider grid demand.

Other trends set to increase the role of smart technology in sustainability include smart charging and the electrification of heat.

Smart charging

Smart charging offers a way for EES technologies, including EV batteries, to act as flexibility for the grid, helping it to cope with demand. Vehicle-to-grid (V2G) and Vehicle-to-home (V2H) charging set-ups will become common in the 2020s, allowing both for support of and independence from the grid.

The electrification of heat

The National Grid is becoming a smart grid. Heat pumps, thermal storage and direct electric heating are being categorized as smart electrical thermal storage (SETS). These offer ways for homes and the grid to operate in harmony, provided the right cabling and ducting is specified at the design stage.

There is no set format for how the smart, energy-efficient home might be configured or what it might contain. Figure 1.3 illustrates one version of the concept. It depicts a connected home that has a smart meter package controlling generators, for example PV, and loads (such as EV), appliances and heating. Notably, the connection to the meter is labelled 'supply/export', reflecting the potential for smart homes with microgeneration or EES to contribute to the grid.

Section 1 – Introduction

Figure 1.3   Illustration of a smart, energy-efficient home (Source: based on a concept from BEAMA)

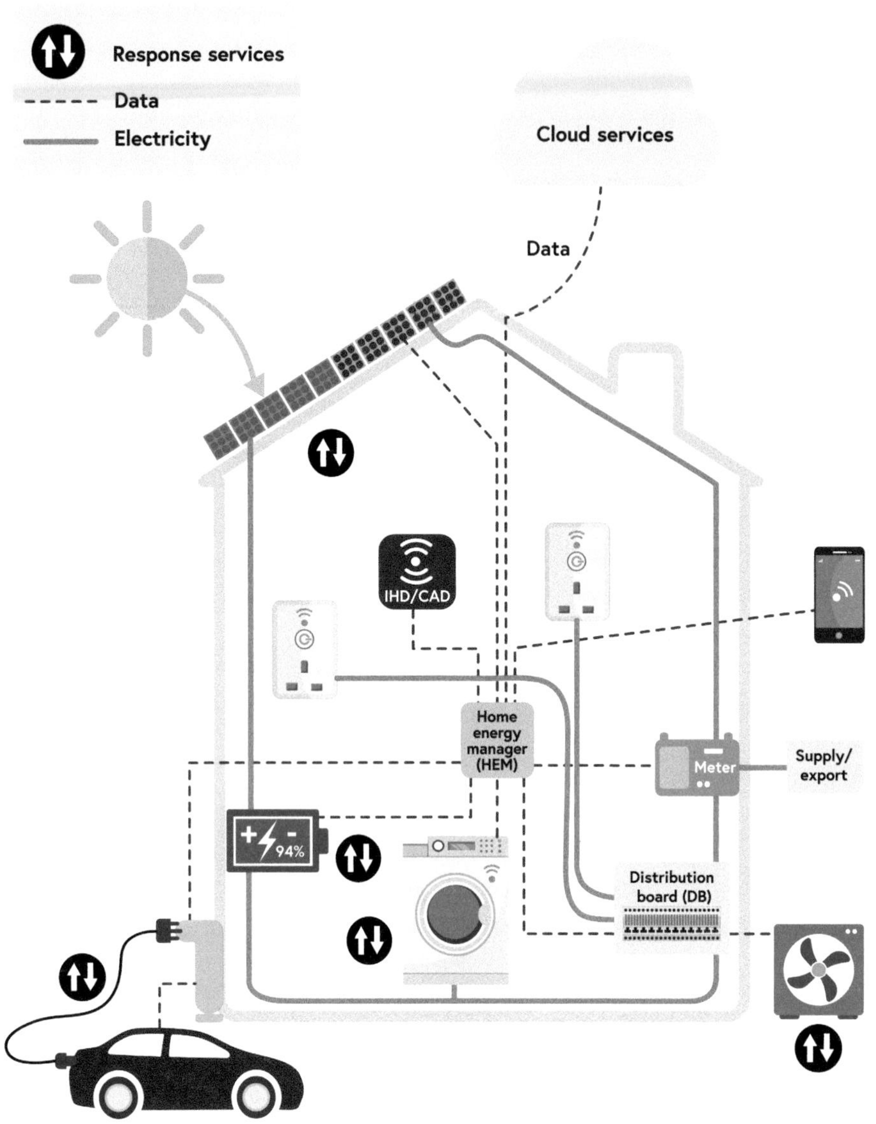

It should be remembered that the proposed UK smart meter package is not a guaranteed route to optimal energy management. Good smart home design should provide infrastructure that allows for energy management in the absence of a smart meter home energy manager (HEM). Strategies for achieving this will be introduced in Section 3.15.

1.6.6   Lighting

Smart possibilities include lights that:

(a) dim and change colour gradually to enhance mood and productivity;

(b) are linked into alarm and alert systems;

(c) simulate presence while occupants are away; and

(d) increase efficiency by only being on when needed.

1.6.7 Infrastructure

There are many manufacturers catering to and expanding on these expectations, and even more ways to design for them. Strategies designed to keep options open include, but are not limited to:

(a) making back boxes for switches deeper (47 mm where possible), to accommodate control gear including wireless modules, and ensuring there is a permanent line, neutral and earth connection in back boxes.

(b) using multicore and/or Ethernet cable (4-twisted pair, for example, CAT5e or CAT6A) to allow for data transmission to luminaires and switch points.

(c) star wiring (explained in more detail later in Section 6 of the Guide).

1.7 Summary

This Section has given an overview of the smart home concept. The rest of this Guide aims to equip the potential installer to handle a smart home project.

This Guide is applicable to domestic installations and small office/home offices (SOHOs). It should be used as a cover-to-cover overview and then as a resource to be dipped into as you progress through a project. It contains explanation, examples, guidance and templates, designed to help you keep a project on track while you focus on the job at hand.

The Sections are organized in the natural order of an installation project, with references to resources you can use placed where they are likely to be needed.

This Guide aims to give you what you need to complete the job without the need to buy other publications. As you progress, you will find areas where your interests or the requirements of a particular project will require further research. Signposts to a directory of further reading contained in Appendix C are therefore embedded in the Guide.

In all electrical design cases, including smart homes, good sense and safety must be prioritized. A designer must consider the *what ifs*. For example: what if smart controls fail due to a fault or a problem with compatibility – should there be a manual override? Experience will inform the answers to this and other typical questions, which this Guide will highlight.

Examples of areas that may require additional research as you develop your smart home practice include:

(a) home network management;

(b) programming;

(c) cyber security;

(d) system integration;

(e) energy management; and

(f) audiovisual (AV) systems.

≡ Section 2

An overview of smart home technology

This Section is extensive, but not exhaustive. It explores and describes the ideas and technologies that are combined to create smart homes.

2.1 Defining 'smart'

Historically, the defining feature of a smart home was that it was automated – and also luxurious and impressive. As Figure 2.1 broadly illustrates, the market and the possibilities have come a long way since the introduction of electric lighting. Smart measures now cover not just automation, but core services like heating, lighting and security. They are also now within the range of modest budgets.

This in turn calls for an improvement in how 'smart' is defined.

Figure 2.1   Transformation of the electric home into the smart home

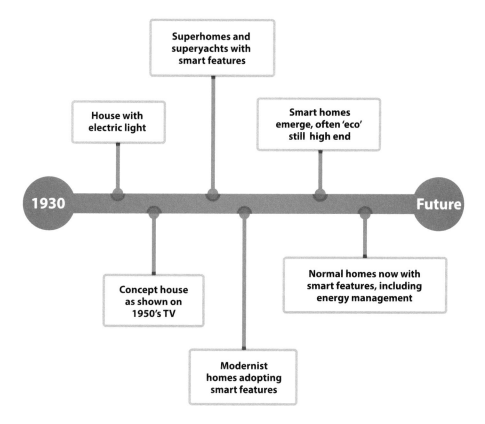

The key distinction of the smart home, compared with the standard home, is the layer of information technology (IT) that sits between the physical system and the user. Software and the processors it runs on create flexibility in the way a connected system can be used.

If that flexibility provides a benefit, then it is a smart measure. For example, if you can set up a switch that previously controlled just your porch light to now arm your new alarm system, that is a smart measure. Another example might be a development of your heating controller to use your phone's location to switch itself on 20 minutes before you get home (geo-mapping).

Section 2 – An overview of smart home technology

Many smart measures and smart devices are designed to be instantly operable (plug and play) and independent of other devices (stand-alone); these are often referred to as 'consumer technology' or 'consumer tech'. The electrical installer's role in smart measure installation typically starts when devices need connections beyond a standard plug and when devices need to be interconnected. At the other end of the spectrum, there is the fully featured bespoke smart home that requires a specialist to consult/design/install and maintain.

This Guide does not attempt to cover the breadth of, or explain in depth, the specific technical details of all smart home possibilities.

This Section gives an overview of how smart homes and in-home smart devices are typically set up at the current time, as well as some consideration of how they might evolve.

This Section will cover:

(a) common elements of a smart home and their topography (how they are laid out);
(b) common smart home topologies (how the elements are connected together);
(c) common smart home software and communication protocols;
(d) examples of smart home setups and how they are implemented; and
(e) examples of smart home products and where they fit into the smart home.

2.2 Common smart home elements

The list of devices and applications that have become smart is growing and will continue to do so. Figure 2.2 shows some common smart home elements.

Figure 2.2   Smart home elements

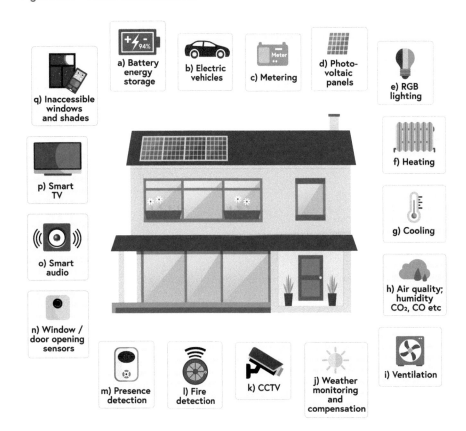

Section 2 – An overview of smart home technology

The applications and functional classes shown in Figure 2.2 can be grouped into categories and expanded upon, as shown here.

Energy

(a) Battery energy storage.
(b) Electric vehicles.
(c) General metering: electricity, fuel, water, etc.
(d) PV panels.

Also consider:

- energy management;
- shading – solar gain; and
- uninterruptible power supply (UPS).

Lighting

(e) Controlled RGB (red, green, blue) lighting:

Also consider:

- shading – light-harvesting/glare prevention;
- dimming;
- presence detection; and
- presence simulation.

Environment

(f) Heating.
(g) Cooling.
(h) Air quality: CO_2, CO, humidity.
(i) Ventilation.
(j) Weather-monitoring and compensation: window/door opening sensors.

Security and boundary

(k) Closed-circuit television (CCTV).
(l) Fire detection.
(m) Presence detection.
(n) Window/door opening sensors.

Also consider:

- presence simulation: lights on/off in an 'away' mode;
- surveillance;
- internet doorbell/intercom/camera;
- door gate opening and closing; and
- window/door opening sensors.

Audiovisual and entertainment

(o) Smart audio.
(p) Smart TV:

Also consider:

- infotainment;
- YouTube;
- streaming music services; and
- radio digital audio broadcasting (DAB).

Section 2 – An overview of smart home technology

Automation/remote operation/assistive technology

(q) Inaccessible windows and shades: access.

Also consider:

- alarm clock;
- window/door opening sensors; and
- alerts to carers.

2.3 User interface (UI)

2.3.1 What defines a smart user interface?

A user interface (UI) is something you use to control equipment.

Most homes have a UI: a traditional thermostat, or even a switch, are examples.

Unlike the thermostat or the switch, however, which will be directly connected to a device it might control, with a smart UI there will be at least one form of separation between the controller and the controlled.

Figure 2.3 illustrates how a switch in a smart home might communicate via IT equipment to a device.

Figure 2.3   UI communicating over IT equipment to a device

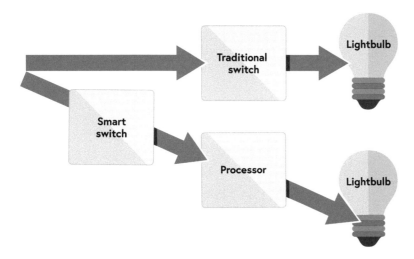

Figure 2.3 could represent a fully featured wired smart home or a simple smart plug. In either case, an IT layer – a processor, or, increasingly likely, a server – will sit between the controller and the controlled device.

Section 2 – An overview of smart home technology

2.3.2 What do smart home UIs look like?

Any combination of the following options can constitute a smart home UI.

Screens

Screens are now a very common UI, owing to the ubiquity of smartphones and tablets that can display UIs by using an app. These devices run on operating systems (OS), for example, Android or Apple iOS, that are strictly maintained by others. This makes good economic sense, in that there is no need to purchase an additional control and the IT maintenance is reduced.

Figure 2.4   A screen-based smart home UI

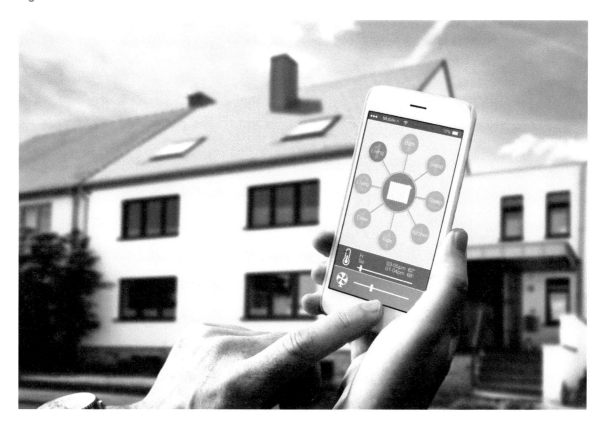

Buttons, dials and levers

Many users prefer something they can really get hold of – or at least touch. Some systems therefore provide hardware and software that can work with 'old-fashioned' devices. Integrating on/off information, as with the light switch and thermostat shown in Figure 2.5, is straightforward. Interpretation of information that is analogue, as with the slide dimmer, or in a programming language specific to that equipment, will be more challenging.

Section 2 – An overview of smart home technology

Figure 2.5   A variety of switches connected to a system

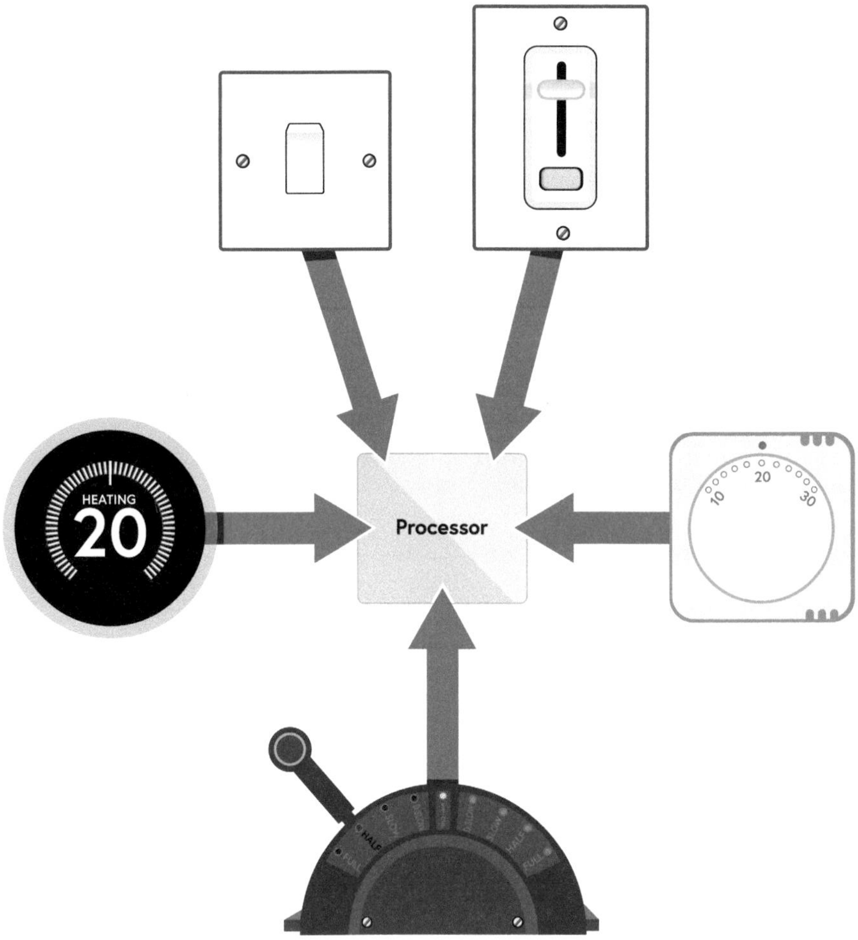

Gesture control

Gesture control is already established in the market, with sensor panels able to detect a swipe direction without the need for touch. A thermostat UI can be mounted on a wall where a traditional switch might otherwise be. It can detect swipe direction, which gives it multi-functionality. Having a digital display, it can easily be purposed for other applications, such as lighting. This sort of control also offers a way to reduce disease transmission by shared-touch controls.

Voice interface

Amazon (Alexa), Google (Google Assistant) and Apple (HomeKit/Siri) have proprietary voice-based interfaces. As these are just three of the most wide-selling and popular voice interfaces, it is very likely that voice control and feedback will become the most numerous UI in future.

Section 2 – An overview of smart home technology

Figure 2.6   Possible topologies of voice-based interfaces

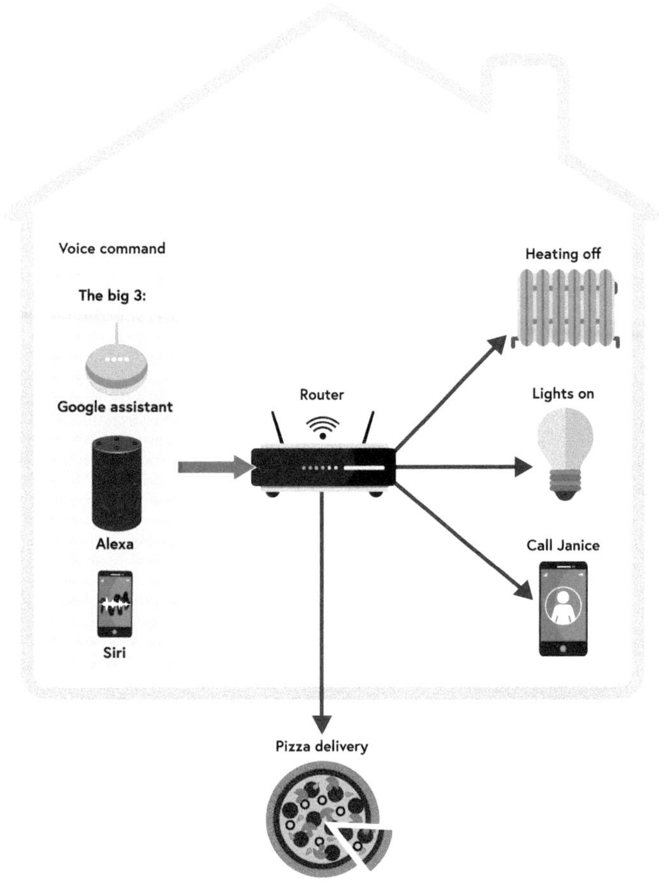

Video-based interface

It is but a short leap from word recognition to image recognition. Number plate and facial recognition are already in use and can be used in smart home systems. Where smart home systems can identify individuals, it becomes possible for the system to tailor its actions to suit the individual. For some years already, we have had cars that adjust to user profiles. Figure 2.7 illustrates one way a smart home might differentiate its response to individuals arriving home.

Section 2 – An overview of smart home technology

Figure 2.7   Differentiated response by video-based interfaces

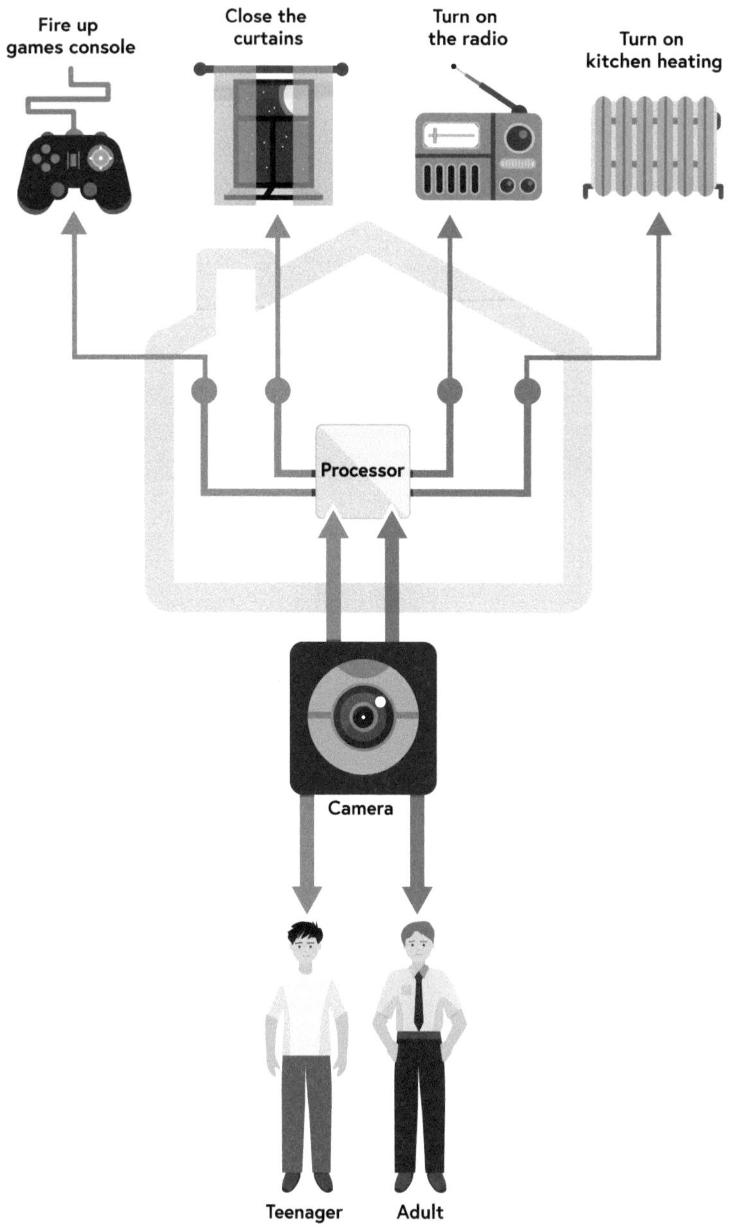

Persona-based interface

AI and machine learning can bypass the need for active control of devices. Smart home system sensors – particularly the video and automated parts – can potentially give platform personas such as Alexa, Google Assistant and Siri a body to inhabit, complete with eyes to see.

The engineer or 'admin' interface

In addition to the everyday UI, there will typically be a means for an engineer to access 'under the bonnet' controls. This might be behind a password or via a separate connection using specific software and possibly hardware tools. This would provide a UI for competent persons to carry out adjustments and maintenance that are best kept away from day-to-day operations, such as software updates or hardware connection information. A trained technician might use this interface to check that devices are communicating properly or running the most up-to-date firmware, which is essential for functionality, but too much information for a day-to-day UI.

2.4   Wired or wireless?

The retrofitted smart home market is bigger than the new-build smart home market and therefore more attractive to manufacturers. Retrofit tends to favour wireless rather than wired devices and this makes it likely that new wireless products will outnumber new wired smart home products. The popularity of wireless seems likely to increase in future. Many householders will buy inexpensive consumer wireless products that claim to do exactly what they need them to do.

2.4.1   When and where should cables be installed?

Typically, a smart installation for a new build property or complete rewire will be predominantly wired.

A retrofit, where the smart measures are the principal component of the project, with material disturbance seen as undesirable, is more likely to be predominantly wireless. It could be augmented by existing wiring, by addition of power-line communication (PLC) plugs, a technology that provides an Ethernet connection between two or more points using the mains power wiring of a house or office.

In many situations, both will be used. An electrical installer should be able to advise householders where there are benefits of hard-wired over wireless smart measures to be considered.

The solution in most cases will be fluid, determined by the needs of the householder and the disturbance to their environment. These two factors: needs and disturbance, must be assessed and balanced. As an electrical installer, you will be accustomed to this situation. As a smart home installer, you have additional things to consider in order to safeguard the effectiveness of the smart measures you are installing. The two factors will be dealt with in more detail in Sections 4 and 5.

Figure 2.8 Wired versus wireless flow diagram

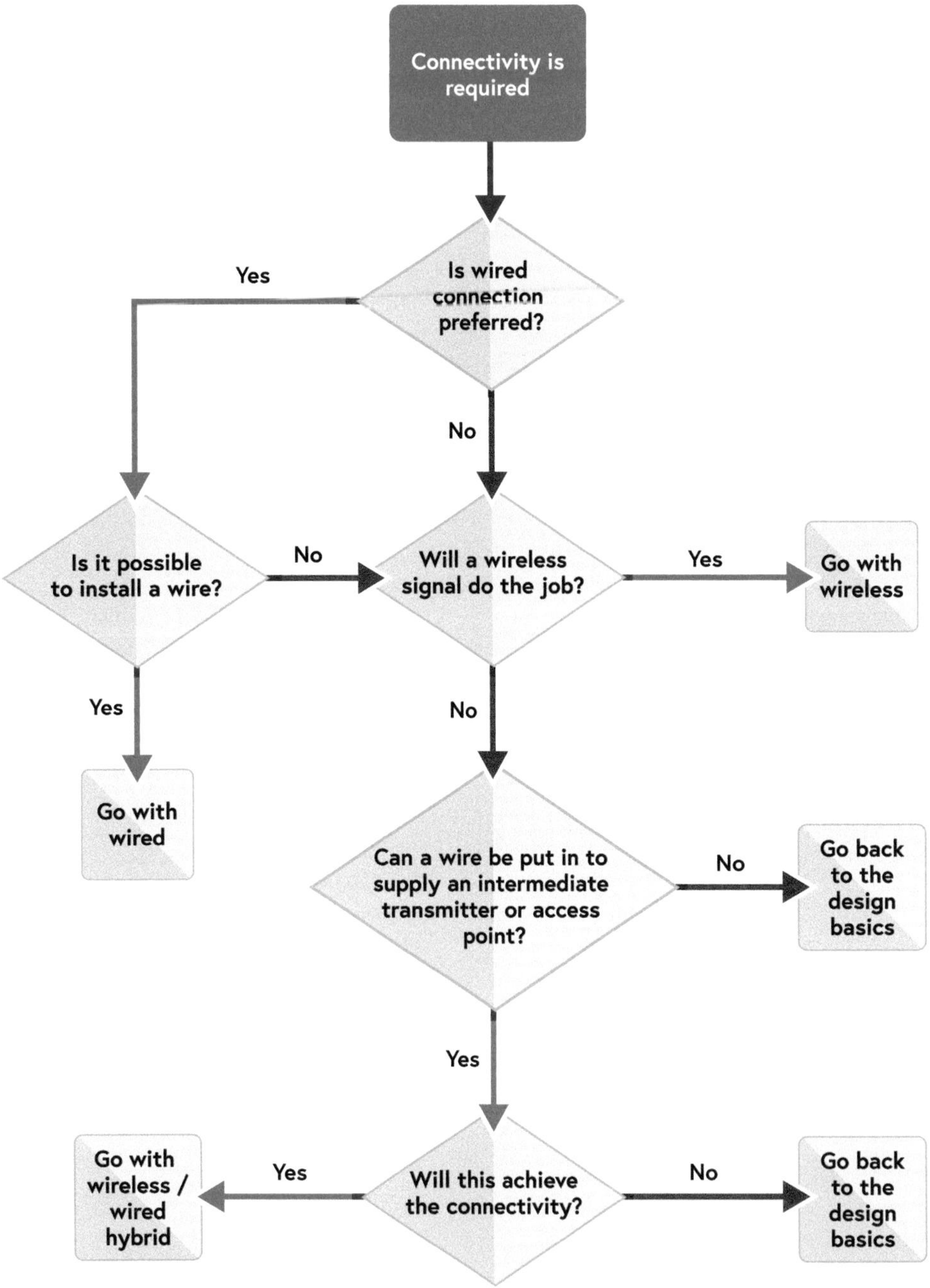

Note: PLC and WiFi devices can be considered. Note that WiFi signal strength can be erratic in many homes unless the smart device is being installed close to the router. Where the signal is weaker, devices may connect on initial installation but fail to sustain the connection. See Section 6.4.1 for further guidance.

2.5 Separated or integrated smartness?

Smart home systems are diverse in design and can be categorized in lots of ways. A key categorization is whether a given smart home system is separated or integrated. Separated systems refer to those that are set apart, distinct or not related: Figure 2.9 depicts some of the separated systems we are accustomed to using in the home. Integrated systems, meanwhile, have various parts or aspects that are linked or co-ordinated: Figure 2.10 shows how the topology changes when systems are integrated.

Section 2 – An overview of smart home technology

2.5.1 Separate

Figure 2.9   Example of separate devices serving functional systems

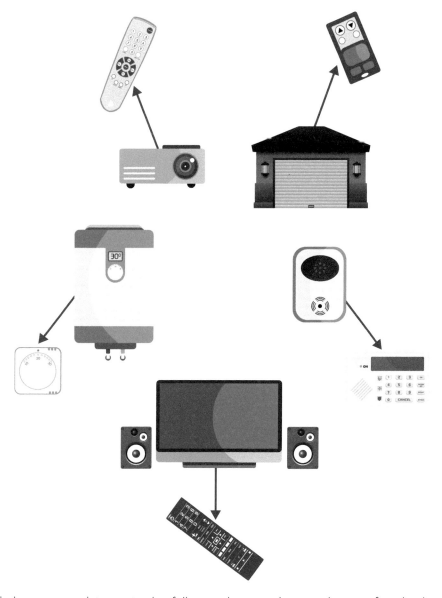

All the separated items in the following list may have a degree of technological sophistication or connectedness that might be described as 'smart':

(a) a garage door that can be opened remotely;

(b) CCTV that can be viewed remotely;

(c) an alarm system that can tell you if a window has been opened;

(d) AV equipment that is connected to the internet and can stream music to your tastes;

(e) fire detection that can message you if it is triggered; and

(f) heating that could fine-tune the efficiency of your central heating to the building fabric, your routine or the local weather.

Section 2 – An overview of smart home technology

2.5.2 Integrated

Integrated smart home systems have something in the middle.

Figure 2.10 Integrated devices connected to a hub

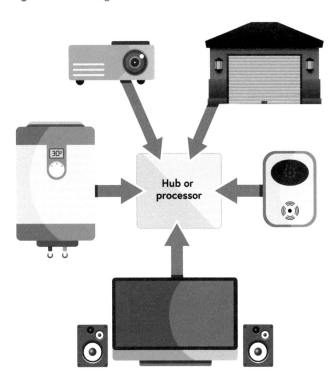

Where there are multiple 'product families' in a home, then the items in that home might be described as 'in-home smart devices', as is the case in Figure 2.9.

Having all functional systems connected back to a single hub in one 'family' creates the possibility that the systems can inform each other. Turning this possibility into a useful reality requires a protocol and platform over which all devices can communicate.

Figure 2.11 illustrates three ways in which an integrated system might be achieved:

1. integrated via a hub: this is the easiest to understand, having a dedicated connection back to a single point.
2. segmented: a scenario that relies on there being technology that can co-ordinate information between the devices. That technology could be a combination of hardware and software.
3. distributed, using cloud/IoT technology. The cloud in this context is where information is held within the internet rather than on local devices. It allows devices to be virtually connected, provided the right software and connectivity is in place.

Section 2 – An overview of smart home technology

Figure 2.11   Three types of integrated home

Integrated via a hub

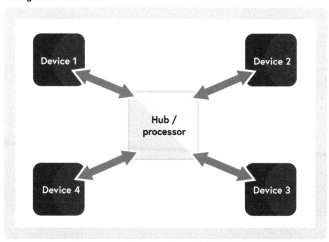

Segmented i.e. more than one hub / product family

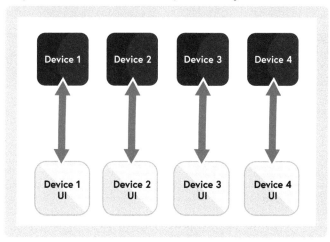

Distributed using cloud / IoT technology

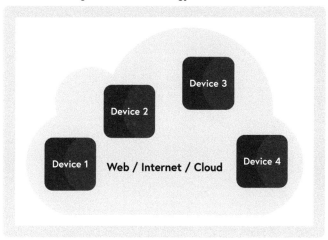

A well designed and integrated smart home will not contain a 'basket of remotes'. As a rule, a smart home designer should, wherever safe and practical, avoid the use of proprietary controls in favour of integrated controls.

2.6 Benefits of connecting systems within a smart home

In most cases, having all devices in a smart home able to communicate with each other is the ideal.

Software is required to achieve this. The environment such software creates is called a 'platform', which is any group of technologies used as a base from which other technologies or software may operate. Amazon's Alexa environment is a famous example of the concept, providing a platform for 'skills' that third-party manufacturers can develop to allow them to work with Alexa.

Having a platform for devices to communicate on creates the possibility that device information can be shared and used to trigger other events, as shown in Figure 2.12. The diagram shows a traditional alarm setup and how, in a smart home, a motion sensor that previously informed an intruder alarm might also inform other systems, to enable a variety of new possibilities:

(a) security: if the alarm is armed, the system could flash lights, open curtains and play loud music, likely to deter intruders;
(b) heating: areas that get irregular use might benefit from having heat-emitters or hot water secondary flow triggered by presence detection carried out by the same sensors used by the alarm; and
(c) lighting: passageways might be enhanced by using the motion sensors to trigger lighting.

Figure 2.12   Comparing the possibilities for traditional (top) and smart (bottom) security systems

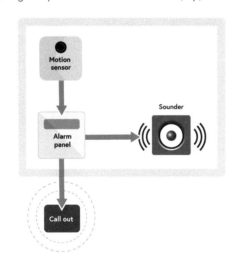

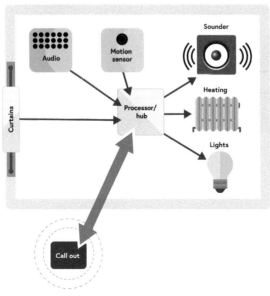

Section 2 – An overview of smart home technology

In addition to enabling additional actions, smart home systems can enable multiple controls. Figure 2.13 shows how shading, such as curtains or blinds, typically controlled by a single button or proprietary remote, might now be controlled by multiple stimuli:

(a) a brightness sensor might be integrated into a motion sensor and used to tell the blinds to adjust to control solar gain, thus regulating temperature or light to avoid glare;

(b) a temperature sensor, in conjunction with a brightness sensor, might be able to judge whether the temperature of the room could be optimized by passively controlling the blinds – letting the blinds up to allow more winter sun in, to save on heating, or letting the blinds down to shield from the summer sun and save on air-conditioning;

(c) a timer scheduler might control the blinds to safeguard privacy or simulate presence while occupants are away; and

(d) an app might allow a householder who is too tired or otherwise unable to push a button to operate the blinds.

Figure 2.13　How shading can be controlled by multiple influences

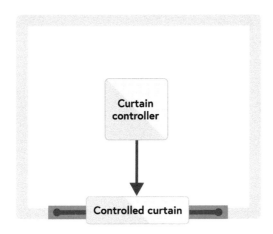

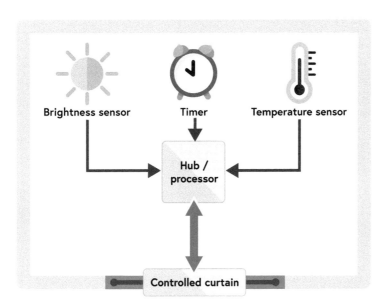

Lighting can be considered in the same way. When arriving home late at night, some householders might want extra lights in the house to come on, in addition to the light in the porch originally specified as the luminaire to be activated by motion. This is not a problem if inputs and outputs are all operating off a single well-designed platform, as shown in Figure 2.14, where all lights are controlled from a single hub.

Figure 2.14 Configuration of additional lights

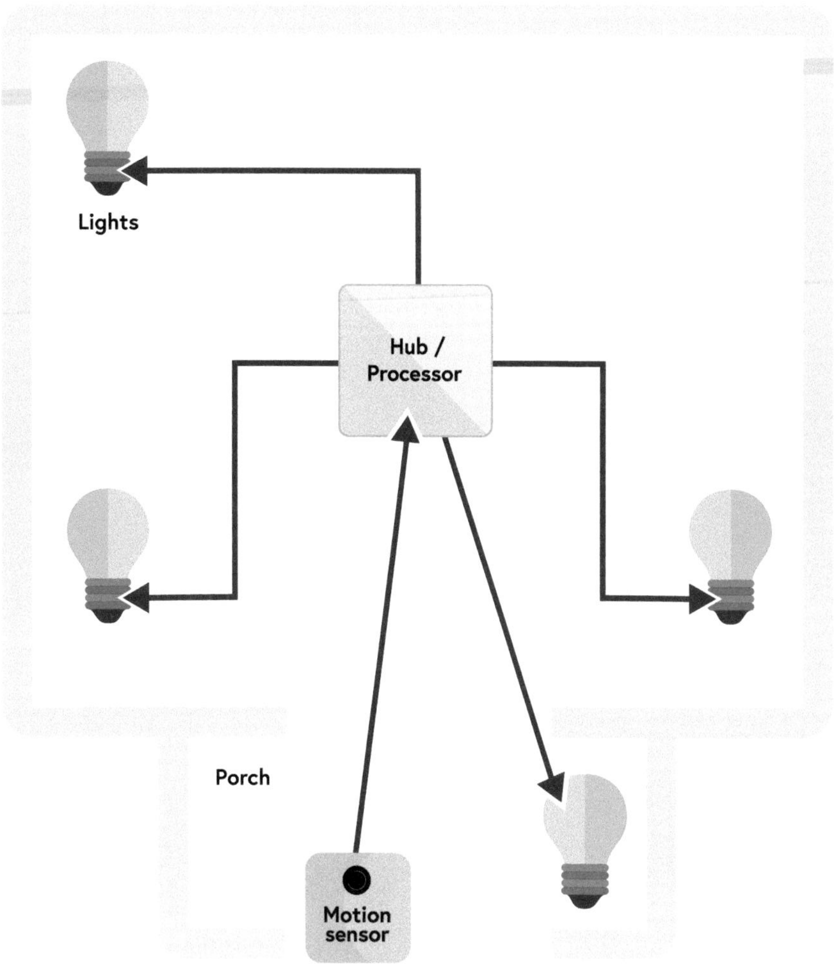

2.7 Interoperability and the cloud

2.7.1 Application programming interface (API)

Historically, making different platform smart home products talk to and co-operate with one another has been a challenging task, undertaken by highly paid specialists known as 'system integrators'. Cloud computing has, however, helped with this situation by creating a virtual space where multiple platforms can share inputs/outputs from connected systems via an application programming interface (API).

An API is a set of programming functions that enable software writers to send and receive commands to and from another device. As an example, If This Then That (IFTTT) an early example of a programming service which can be used to connect devices over the internet: an API might allow an IFTTT device to react to inputs from a google Nest thermostat. Figure 2.15 illustrates a situation where a device could trigger lighting in response to a fire alarm – which could be useful if residents have impaired hearing.

Section 2 – An overview of smart home technology

Figure 2.15   Example of IFTTT

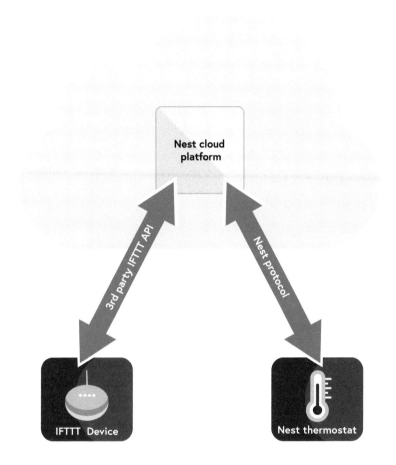

Section 2.5.2 discusses product families. The cloud has the potential to make all internet-connected devices interoperable: able to exchange and make use of information even if they are made by different manufacturers. Clearly, integrated systems have a huge advantage over separated systems, as the whole becomes greater than the sum of the parts and the householder gets a better smart home. Many manufacturers have already seen the potential in this philosophy and acted on it.

2.7.2   Internet of Things (IoT)

The IoT is not a platform, but a description of some features of connected devices – broadly speaking, the ability to communicate, to some degree, with other IP devices.

A commonly agreed approximate number of IoT devices in 2020 is 20 billion, which is a lot of devices and potentially represents a lot more traffic on the internet.

Section 2 – An overview of smart home technology

Figure 2.16   Examples of IoT end-device products

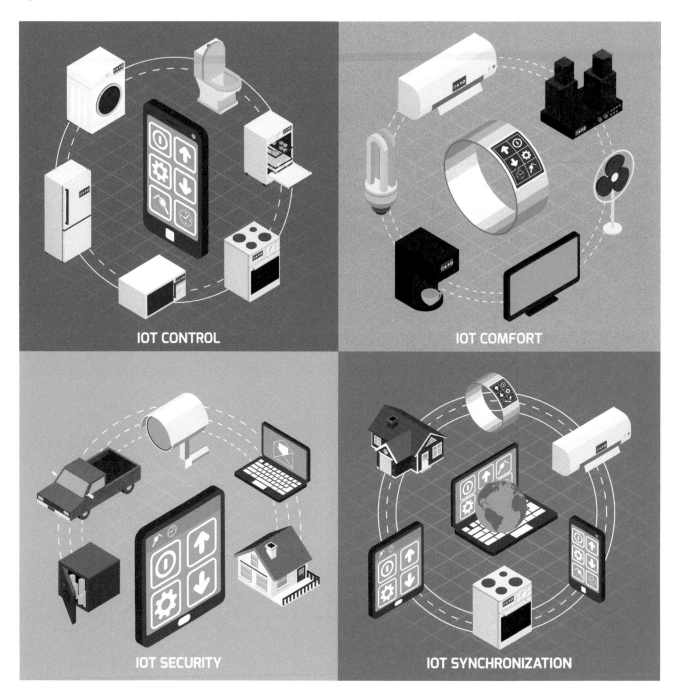

Advantages and disadvantages of the IoT

IoT advocates focus on its convenience and potential to link up everything, everywhere.

Critics, meanwhile, focus on issues to do with privacy, security and resilience. What if we all 'swap over' to the IoT and it is somehow disabled – for example, by hacking, or an infrastructure failure like a power cut? Not all IoT devices are internet-dependent, and nor are we all likely to 'swap over', but this remains a concern for many.

Section 2 – An overview of smart home technology

For the electrical installer looking at the smart home industry, the IoT is a new class of connectivity. With organizations like Amazon, Apple and Google backing it, it is likely to become common to the industry.

Some electrical contractors are also wary of the IoT, much as factory workers might fear the development of robots or as small shops might have concerns about the growth of supermarkets. The case here is more complicated, but it should be remembered that one IoT device might control a multitude of non-IoT devices, which require substantial cabled connections. The electrical installer who understands how this all works is still very much in the picture in an IoT future.

2.7.3 DIY interoperability

Some electrical installers will wish to take on system integration themselves. APIs can enable programmers to interface two separate devices to enable communications between them (interoperability).

Options for this include:

(a) IFTTT;
(b) Amazon Alexa Skill Blueprints;
(c) Apple HomeKit;
(d) experimenting with the IoT yourself, perhaps through a Raspberry Pi; and
(e) writing your own APIs or 'applets' (note that this is an advanced option and should probably be deferred until you are secure with the basics).

Until, and probably after, you become a master-coder, the following simple interoperability rules should be followed, to avoid expensive mistakes:

(a) read all the information on any devices you want to make interoperable.
(b) do the devices say that they are interoperable? Many manufacturers have a strict 'works with' accreditation system with its own logo that should be displayed. Act accordingly.
(c) with smart homes, a very high degree of what is possible is determined by the purchase, so do not assume otherwise.
(d) always test any new products for interoperability before recommending them to customers.

2.8 Smart home information and processing

2.8.1 Where to look and why

Different systems handle processing and information differently. Some might keep all information and processing ability in a box in the centre of the smart home, while others keep it all outside. Many others adopt a 'happy medium' approach.

A householder might never need to know which bit of the smart measure that they have adopted does the 'thinking'. However, when an electrical installer comes to design a smart system, they should find this out before specifying, as it may have implications.

To ensure that systems work as required and are not overstretched, an electrical installer needs to consider where in the system:

(a) decisions are made;
(b) data is sent; and
(c) data is stored.

Section 2 – An overview of smart home technology

There are two main areas for consideration

1. data traffic and volume; and
2. resilience and critical safety.

Intelligence might be located:

(a) in the cloud;
(b) within the connected devices;
(c) within a processor or node; or
(d) may be distributed.

Option (d) offers the most system resilience, as it is less likely that intelligence will be disconnected. Where there is uncertainty about resilience, manufacturers should be approached for guidance.

Figure 2.17   Example of where intelligence is located (a-d)

(a) smart home and cloud with 'brain' in the cloud;
(b) smart home with many little brains in lots of smaller devices;
(c) smart home with brain in the hub; and
(d) different sized brains in various places.

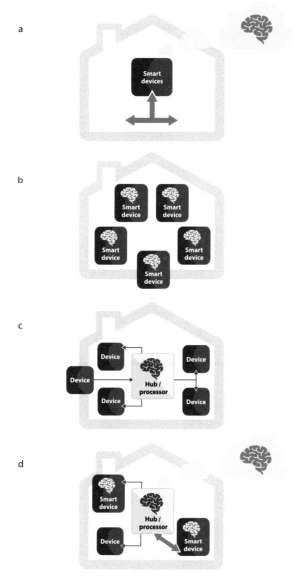

Section 2 – An overview of smart home technology

2.8.2 Data traffic

Smart devices communicate and sometimes store information. Most of that information is digitized: on/off or 1s and 0s, as opposed to analogue/variable signals. There is a limit to the rate at which digital information can be sent through any medium such as copper wire, optical fibre or WiFi. This limit is usually referred to as the bandwidth – the amount of data that can be sent in a given length of time, usually megabits per second (Mbps).

Figure 2.18 shows a more densely populated version of Figure 1.1, where we considered how communication is increasingly passed through the home router. Most modern homes will look more like Figure 2.18 and that results in a lot of information over the home network.

Figure 2.18   Traffic-creating devices

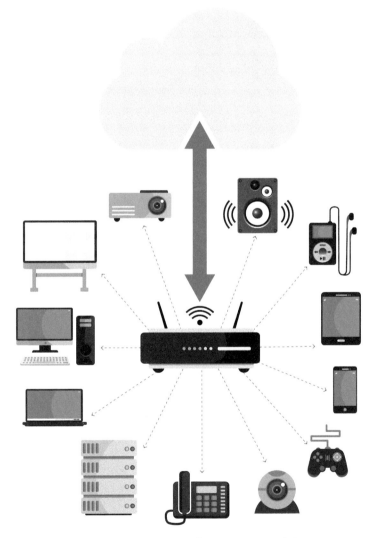

It is possible to exceed the data-capacity of equipment and this can cause it to malfunction. A designer should consider the bandwidth requirements of devices to be installed and match this to the capacity of other equipment, such as cables and storage.

Some devices send and receive more data than others. Elements that will significantly increase traffic include:

(a) AV multi-media; and
(b) video and audio surveillance – particularly if this is not processed or compressed.

Section 2 – An overview of smart home technology

This reflects the detailed and constantly varying information relayed in video signals. Conversely, a connection to a window to register when it is open and closed will use very little data by comparison, as there are only two states (open/closed) and the variation between those states will be infrequent.

Camera surveillance can be a heavy bandwidth burden and the consequences of its failure are potentially expensive, for example, if insurance cover is compromised. It is advisable to take time to make sure infrastructure is adequate.

Figure 2.19   CCTV and bandwidth

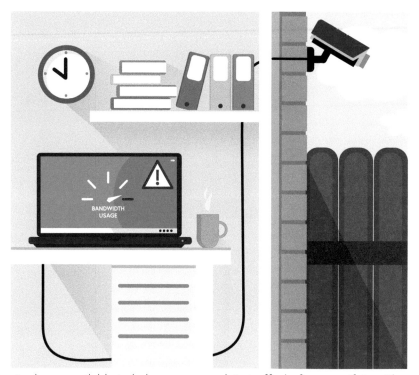

Online tools are available to help you assess data traffic before specifying. The screenshot in Figure 2.20 is representative of a reseller's website and can tell you how choices affect bandwidth and storage options.

Figure 2.20   Online data estimation tool

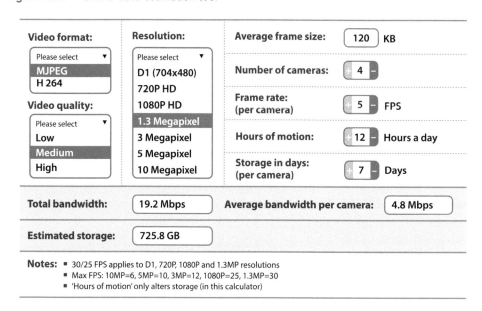

Section 2 – An overview of smart home technology

Dedicated server data

While IoT devices are becoming increasingly dominant, not all systems use the home area network (HAN). These systems are unlikely to need anything like the bandwidth required for AV.

Care should be taken, however, to ensure that data does not accumulate. Overkill on data-capture, for example data-logging temperature, humidity and light levels at 1-second intervals in a 15-zone home, might not break the smart home network instantly, but could affect system performance over time.

When designing, you should determine the likely level of traffic that will pass through the HAN or smart home network. In any network, data adds up and cables and network equipment (switches and storage) that are 'overstretched' can lead to problems and even system failure.

To assess traffic, you need to understand which components are communicating and at what rate. Manufacturers' specifications are the best source of this information. Figure 2.21 gives a guide to some common elements.

Figure 2.21   Examples of various devices and their bandwidth

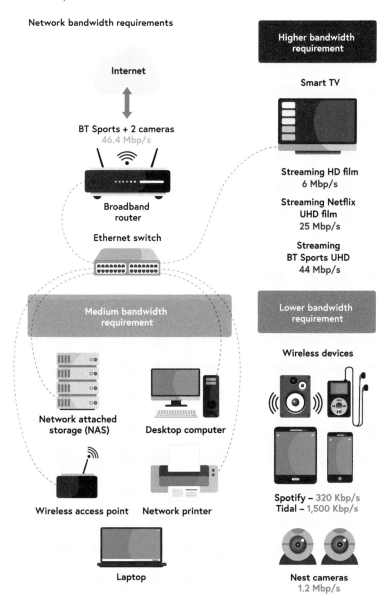

2.9 Software and protocols

Figure 2.22 illustrates a way in which connected systems like smart homes can stack up, from the physical environment (for example, rooms) and containment at the bottom, to the UI, which sits at the top.

Figure 2.22 Illustration of the layers in smart home systems

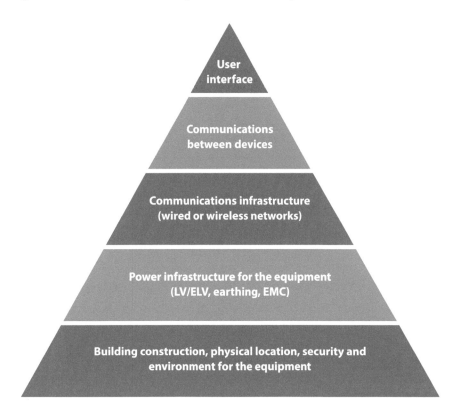

The top three layers of Figure 2.22 comprise what is commonly referred to as a 'platform'. This can have physical and software elements. The concept is fluid, but a smart home installer can think of it as the bundle of technology that makes the connectedness work.

An electrical installer progressing into the smart home industry does not necessarily need all the details of this, but does need broadly to understand how the software and physical elements of a system relate to each other:

(a) the bottom layers (4 and 5) will be familiar to electrical installers.
(b) layer 3 is more specialized, involving work with data networks. Some will have already broached this and signposts to training can be found in Appendix C.
(c) layer 2 is the signals, which will be in a set protocol if the system is to work, and the software.
(d) layer 1 is the part that the system users interact with.

The client will be interested in the UI (layer 1) and the elements it controls (layer 5). The smart home installer's job is to ensure that the infrastructure in between is coherent.

Software is central to ensuring coherence and is dealt with in more detail below.

Section 2 – An overview of smart home technology

2.9.1 Software: proprietary or open source?

Proprietary software

Proprietary software is software that is sold with the product. Sometimes known as 'closed protocol', you will not have access to the code to adapt it for your own systems. This software is owned or licensed by the manufacturer and should be maintained and developed by them. Its identity and branding will be set and controlled.

Examples of proprietary software include:

(a) Microsoft Windows; and
(b) Trend IQ, a well-established commercial building management system (BMS) software product.

Open source software

This is software that has been developed and released into the world free of charge.

Typically, the original code will be taken up by developers and turned into something that matches an application (smart home systems can be described as an application). It can be confusing to trace the origins of open source applications, as there is no strict control on identity and branding.

Examples of open source software include:

(a) Linux, which can be run on personal computers (PCs) and a range of devices, including Raspberry Pi; and
(b) Alexa Skills, which can be used to configure IoT devices.

2.9.2 Is one better than the other?

Proprietary software can be convenient, but it can also be restrictive. Software development costs money and manufacturers understandably want a return on their investment. They might design their software to favour their own products.

Open source software is typically less convenient, because it usually has to be adapted, but is less restrictive, because the distributors design it to be adapted.

A happy compromise might be 'shared source' software. Such software might be developed and maintained by a guild of manufacturers, developers and electrical installers, where there is a 'buy in' for all parties. One example of shared software is that produced by the KNX Alliance: an electrical installer would typically pay for training on this, then for a KNX software licence. In return, they would have access to a range of regulated, accredited and, hopefully, well-supported materials and resources.

In reality, proprietary and open source software are blending. They might be blended within a device or system, for example, with some proprietary functional software running over standard communications protocols. The trend towards the IoT and globalized connectivity seems likely to discriminate against 'island' mentality software that promotes reliance on its own product family. However, with organizations like Amazon, Google, Apple and Samsung competing, we should not rule out the possibility that a dominant brand will emerge.

The important thing to remember is that any of the options (proprietary, open and shared) has the potential to be excellent or disastrous – and everything in between.

Electrical installers are advised always to investigate software before investing in the products on which it runs. Certainly, elements such as the cost and quality of training and the support on offer after installation should be confirmed. It is worth looking at forums or review websites to pick up feedback and advice from those who have previously used the software. Table 2.1 provides a list of questions that could be asked about smart home software.

Section 2 – An overview of smart home technology

Table 2.1   Software checklist

Question	Answer
Is training required to programme the system?	
Do the manufacturers offer software training?	
How long is the training?	
What does the training cost?	
When and how often does training happen?	
How often do software updates happen?	
How will training be updated as the software is updated?	
Is there email/web support for the software?	
Is there email/web support for the hardware?	
Are there reviews for the software?	
Is it possible to access a demo version of the configuration software?	
Is it possible to access a demo version of the UI?	

2.9.3   What is a communication protocol?

Broadly, a communication protocol is the part of the system that allows communication between devices. Referring back to Figure 2.22, it would sit between the UI and the communications infrastructure.

The switch in Figure 2.23 represents the simplest possible protocol: open and closed. Smart homes commonly use this protocol to create two states you will be familiar with: on and off.

Figure 2.23   A simple smart home protocol in practice

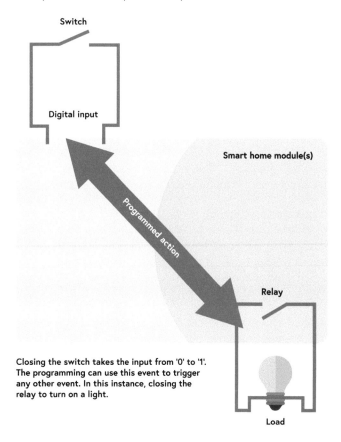

Closing the switch takes the input from '0' to '1'. The programming can use this event to trigger any other event. In this instance, closing the relay to turn on a light.

Section 2 – An overview of smart home technology

In 1836 Henry Morse invented a code that allowed those states (open/closed/on/off) to be translated into language. All IT communication protocols are variations on this theme. 'Ons' and 'offs' have become 1s and 0s and these have been translated into a variety of 'alphabets', which arguably started with the American Standard Code for Information Interchange (ASCII) codes.

With regard to IT systems, communication between devices requires that the devices agree on the format of the data. The set of rules defining a format is the communication protocol.

2.9.4 What are communication protocols used for?

The list below outlines some of the most common examples of the use of communication protocols:

(a) WiFi, also known as IEEE 802.11: dominant for retrofit smart measures. It provides wireless communications back to a router or similar device. It may be augmented by wireless access points (WAPs) or PLC Ethernet.
(b) RS-485: a physical layer used by numerous protocols, including Modbus, DMX and many that are manufacturer-specific.
(c) RS-232: a Standard originally introduced in 1960 for the serial communication transmission of data.
(d) Zigbee: an open protocol for mesh-networks, notably used by UK smart meters. Limited to specific platforms, without much interoperability.
(e) Z-wave: a wireless radio frequency (RF) protocol.
(f) transmission control protocol/internet protocol (TCP/IP): how most devices on the internet find each other.
(g) 1-wire: provides low-speed data, signalling and power over a single conductor. In practice, there is usually more than one conductor.
(h) digital addressable lighting interface (DALI): a system to make lights individually addressable.
(i) Bluetooth: only for short distance, for example, for local audio.
(j) Bluetooth low energy (BLE): for close-range lower-rate data transmission between devices.
(k) OpenTherm: a protocol to more efficiently co-ordinate many modern boilers and thermostats.

One or two from this list should be familiar to you and give you a sense of where communication protocols sit – in between devices, allowing them to communicate with each other.

It is useful for the electrical installer to recognize what a protocol is, so that they can place it in context. Smart home manufacturers may offer a range of hardware add-ons and software patches to enable you to integrate devices that use a certain protocol.

A good example concerns utility metering. M-Bus is by far the most popular protocol for linking to meters. If your business model is based around energy management, this may be one protocol that you might wish to take some time to gain, or hire, proficiency with.

2.10 Infrastructure for smart home systems

This Section illustrates how smart home installation may be different physically to 'traditional' installations, with the focus predominantly on wired systems. Remember that wired systems might be designed to serve as a backbone for wireless and distributed systems through WiFi and other proprietary signals.

In general, the following statements will hold true:

(a) power circuits will stay much the same; but
(b) everything else will need a design rethink.

Section 2 – An overview of smart home technology

2.10.1 Cabling

The first thing to understand is that in a smart installation, more cables will run from a central point, as opposed to linking on from other cables.

Figure 2.24 shows very simplistically how the cabling for a smart home (in the lower diagram) differs from standard wiring (in the upper diagram). Anything that needs to be controlled individually should have its own cable back to the 'board'. Switches in a smart home are not 'looped in' to specific devices, but are instead wired back to the board or hub/processor.

Figure 2.24 Smart versus traditional wiring for lighting

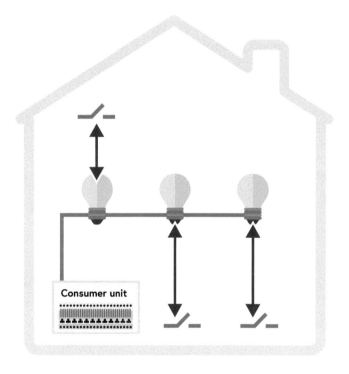

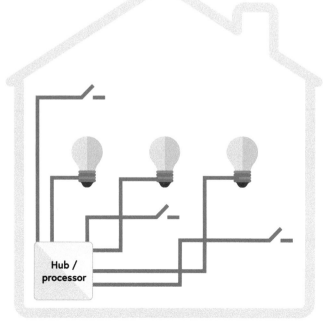

Section 2 – An overview of smart home technology

Figure 2.25 illustrates a greater variety of devices, but the same principle for cabling, in which everything goes back to the hub. This allows for more flexibility in control, which will be explored in more detail in Section 6 of the Guide.

Figure 2.25   Smart wiring for other functional systems

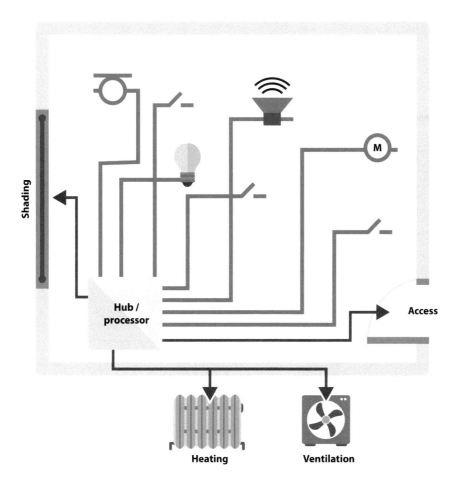

2.10.2 The hub/processor

The traditional domestic electrical installation, as shown in Figure 2.26, has the functional systems distributed and separate. The only connection between these elements would be a shared live feed, usually via a fused connection outlet or socket-outlet, which would be fed from the consumer unit (or distribution board (DB), as it shall be referred to in this Guide).

Figure 2.26   System topology in a traditional home

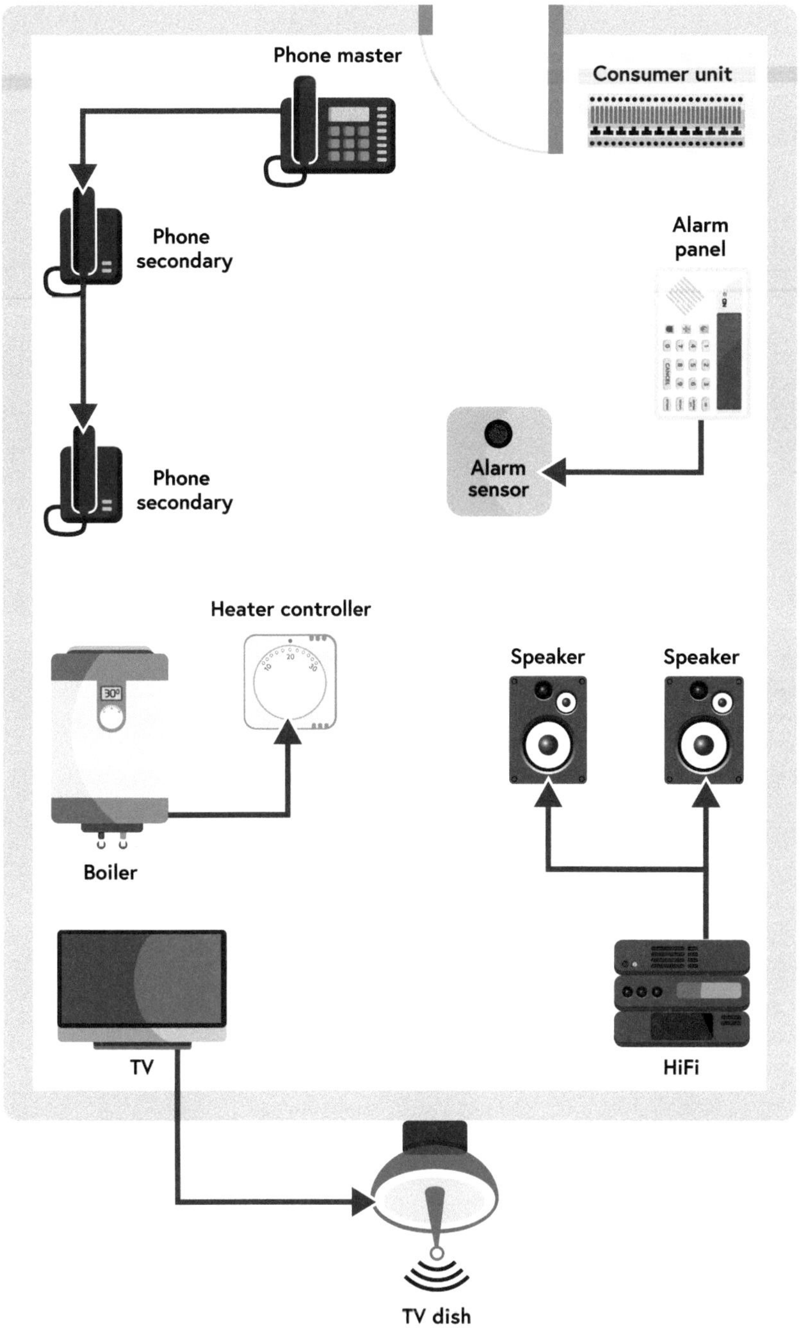

This lack of interconnection is not ideal for a smart home, where we need connectedness. Best practice for infrastructure in a smart home is to set up a hub/processor, as shown in Figure 2.27. The common name for such a hub is a smart home head end (SHHE), also known as a low voltage head end (LVHE) or even an extra-low voltage head end (ELVHE). For brevity, this Guide will use the term 'head end' (HE).

Section 2 – An overview of smart home technology

Figure 2.27 The HE at the centre of everything

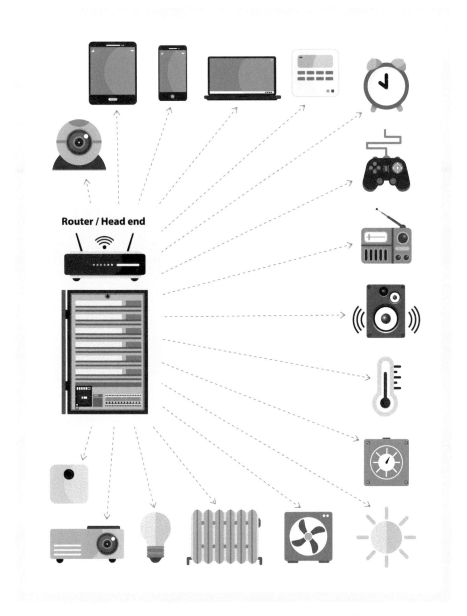

Figure 2.27 represents the classical HE and the smart home format that most requires the services of an electrical installer. It shows an area to which all electrical and electronic devices are wired back, and from which devices are monitored and controlled.

The primary HE should be where incoming services, for example, TV, satellite and broadband/telephone services, are terminated within the home. It is also where cables to rooms should be terminated, ideally into patch panels, where appropriate.

Secondary HEs, effectively sub-distribution points, may be required where cabling considerations dictate.

Not all smart homes will have a recognizable HE. For example, for those with IoT or stand-alone smart devices, the HE may be a box by the router, or in the cloud.

Any configuration of equipment is possible and acceptable, provided it is safe and meets expectations.

Section 2 – An overview of smart home technology

An HE is a hub for all the systems in a home, as shown in Figure 2.28.

Figure 2.28   HE at the centre of smart home systems

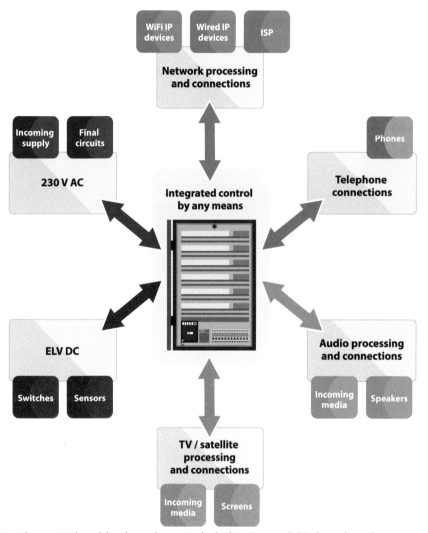

Notice that switch cables have been included in Figure 2.28, but that they are not grouped with 230 V cabling. This is because they are not typically 230 V devices.

2.10.3 Structured cabling

Many new buildings are having structured cabling built into their fabric in anticipation of smart technology being installed ('future-readying'). This typically takes the form of additional Ethernet cable to carry internet signals to entertainment areas. This can add value to a home even without the entertainment systems being installed.

As an electrical installer, you will be accustomed to installing data cable for systems including telephone, Ethernet, video and alarms. These will probably have been tackled one at a time, in separation. A smart home, however, needs a different approach, because:

(a) there will be more data cables; and
(b) the data cables take on a different role, in which they are central to the operation of the building.

The approach required to create coherent safe wiring systems in the smart home application is called 'structured cabling'.

Section 2 – An overview of smart home technology

Structured cabling is a complete system of cabling and related hardware, providing an all-inclusive communications infrastructure. It should serve as wide a range of uses as can be envisaged for the installation. It should not be device-dependent, but rather a backbone on which devices sit.

Figure 2.29 Structured organization of cabling (Adapted with permission from material provided by CEDIA)

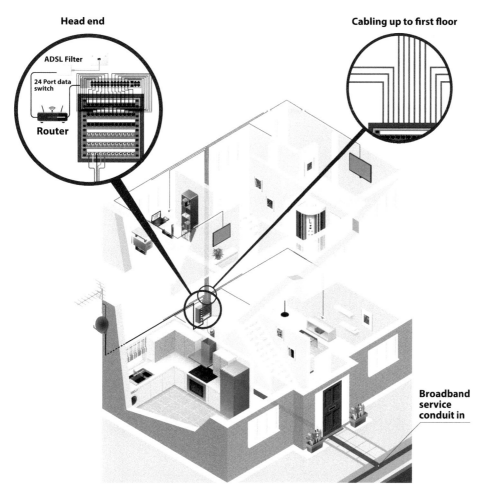

This illustration shows how wired ethernet might be distributed using structured cabling from a head end. Similar configurations for additional systems would run in parallel according to manufacturers guidance and create the structured cabling infrastructure.

This Guide does not attempt to instruct an electrical installer on the methods and theory of structured cabling. Books and training courses on the subject are referenced in Appendix C. Figure 2.30 shows the standard the industry expects on the right, and the standard you are likely to achieve without careful planning or training on the left.

Figure 2.30   Unstructured (left) versus structured cabling (right)

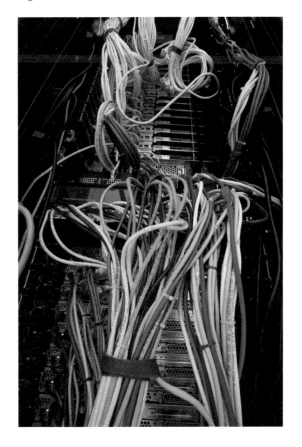 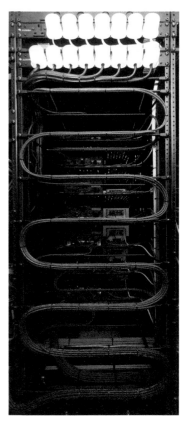

2.10.4 Sensors

To design smart homes, it is necessary to adopt the broadest possible definition of a sensor. The following provides a starting point.

A sensor is a device that detects or measures a physical property and records, indicates or otherwise responds to it. Consideration of sensors, whether wired or wireless, in smart homes is a good opportunity to align your thinking to the differences and the possibilities as you make the transition from traditional design.

The word 'sensor' implies electronics and sophistication and probably a probe of some sort. Not many people would include the word 'switch' if they were asked to write a list of five sensors, but a smart home designer should, because:

(a) a switch will probably be connected back to the same place and in the same manner as all the other sensors;

(b) switch locations that previously contained buttons and rockers might now contain more sophisticated devices, such as gesture-based sensors;

(c) a switch plate might contain other sensors, for example, for presence detection, temperature or humidity; and

(d) a switch is, by definition, a sensor, as it senses the operator's desire to perform an action.

Smart home switches might be multi-functional, as in the left example in Figure 2.31, or application-specific, as in the right example.

Section 2 – An overview of smart home technology

Figure 2.31   Options available with a switch (Reproduced by permission of ABB)

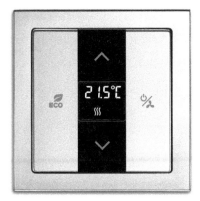 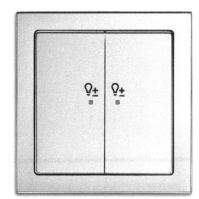

As you progress with smart home design, you should remember that anything can be measured. Consider, at the extreme, that organizations such as Facebook and Amazon have developed algorithms designed to assess mood, based on web-browsing patterns. Facial recognition can now also be used to attempt to gauge mood. This might not be a strictly 'physical' property, but it raises the question of how far we might be from a house that adjusts music or lighting according to mood. Such a house might select a cheering film to stream, or order a tub of your favourite ice cream to be delivered to your door, by drone of course.

2.11   Summary

In this Section, we have considered the central ideas and technologies found in smart homes. There is a good deal of information to be retained and balanced by the smart home installer. For ease, the strands could be broken down into the following categories:

(a) devices;
(b) virtual elements, for example, software; and
(c) infrastructure, for example, structured cabling.

The challenge, going forward, is to be able to combine the most appropriate equipment to match the needs of the smart home client. Section 4 addresses this challenge.

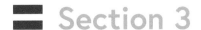

How smart home products are applied

This Section introduces the most common components with which you, as a smart home installer, are likely to work. It is not exhaustive and does not describe the standard electrical components that are needed but with which an electrical installer will already be familiar.

3.1 Smart home HE modules

DIN rail-mounted modules are still the most common format for wired smart home controls.

Figure 3.1   Typical DIN-mounted module (Reproduced by permission of Loxone)

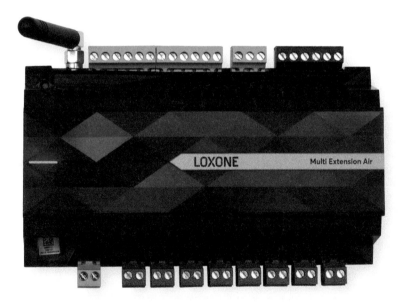

3.2 WiFi and PLC

Sometimes, a single router is not enough and structured cabling will be required to extend the network. Anyone who has used WiFi will be familiar with the frustration of dropping signal when WiFi roaming or 'handoff' has not been properly provisioned. This extract from Section 6.8.7 of the IET *Code of Practice for Connected Systems Integration in Buildings* describes the difference between wireless repeaters and WAP:

> *There are two ways of increasing WiFi coverage: wireless repeaters or additional WAPs.*
> *A wireless repeater (also known as a wireless extender) connects to the existing wireless network, acting as another device on that network, and then uses its own radio to re-transmit the wireless data. When using a wireless repeater be aware that data rate is therefore divided (because the bandwidth is shared between transmitting and receiving). The portion of the network bandwidth available to devices that are connected to the repeater will be limited by the portion of the overall WiFi bandwidth that the repeater shares with all other WiFi devices that are connected to the original access point.*
> *A supplementary WAP does not give rise to this problem; however, it will need its own wired connection to the backbone of the Ethernet network and own power supply (which could be PoE) in order to create a new 'fresh' WiFi network in its local area.*

Figure 3.2   Different topologies of WiFi repeaters and access points

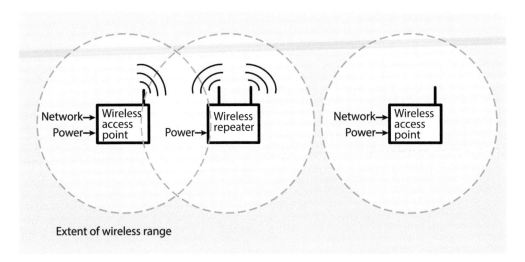

Where appropriate, a PLC plug, as mentioned in Section 2.4.1 and shown in Figure 3.3, can be used to create a WAP WiFi zone. Plugs should always be paired and should not be used in plug and play mode, so that encryption is invoked and private data will not be visible on a neighbour's wiring. Concerns that some PLC devices create undesirable interference have been addressed to some extent. Dedicated Ethernet cabling is undoubtedly better, but PLC can be a huge enabler where it is not possible to run new cables. Signposts to further information on PLC can be found in Appendix C.

Figure 3.3   A PLC WAP using a standard plug socket

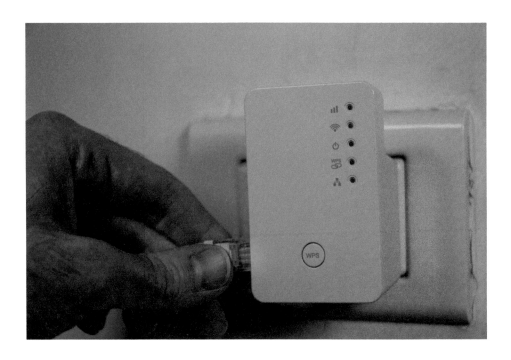

3.3   Stand-alone consumer tech

Some consumer tech products do one job very well and can be more cost-effective than a wired/HE approach. Typically, consumer tech will need a 13 A socket-outlet with a WiFi and/or cable connection to the router, which the electrical installer may be required to install as well. For example, the camera shown in Figure 3.4 is supplied with its own plug/power supply and cable and readily connects to the HAN via WiFi.

Figure 3.4   Stand-alone consumer-tech camera

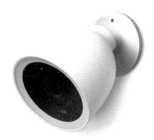

3.4   Smart appliances

Smart appliances are still less common than traditional appliances, but they are trending rapidly. Possible means of connection include:

(a) wired Ethernet (generally found on smart TVs and some large heating appliances, such as boilers);
(b) WiFi (the most common);
(c) Zigbee/Z-Wave; and
(d) PLC, which can enable connection via an RJ45 socket on the appliance even where there is no Ethernet, but only a mains socket.

WiFi is currently the favoured connection, so the smart home design should ensure that WiFi coverage is adequate to support multiple devices in all locations in which they might be found.

Zigbee is a specialized wireless signal, used by the UK smart meter package.

Wired Ethernet points are necessary to connect to a smart appliance that has an Ethernet (RJ45) socket. Remember that these could also serve to connect access points for WiFi or Zigbee if they were required to do so later.

Figure 3.5   Smart white goods

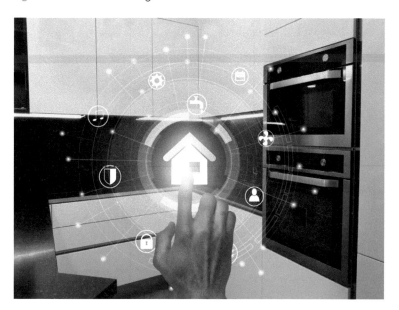

3.5   A smart or wireless plug

Not all locations can be wired to, and no design can anticipate every requirement. A wirelessly controlled smart plug can therefore be invaluable for delivering on/off functionality. For example, a new glass cabinet might need lighting: a nearby socket could be used to supply and switch lights via a smart socket, as pictured in Figure 3.6. Some smart sockets have added functionality, such as energy measurement and temperature sensing.

Note: The device described above can come in the form of a plug-in adaptor or be part of a socket plate.

Figure 3.6   Smart socket/plate (Reproduced by permission of Scolmore)

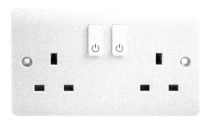

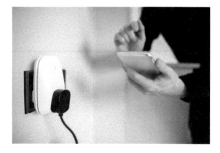

3.6 Motion sensors

The passive infrared (PIR) or, in some cases, microwave sensors found in standard lighting and security systems can be merged in a smart home system to provide information for any number of functions, as shown in Figure 2.2. They can be installed on any surface, in order to achieve the best view of the zone. Intruder alarm sensors that fit neatly in corners are often used, but the installer should bear in mind that a sensor that informs other functional groups as well as an intruder alarm might need to be positioned differently. Positioning will be covered in more detail in Section 7.7.2.

A typical smart home configuration of motion sensors would allocate one motion sensor per room (large rooms and open-plan houses will vary this requirement). Wall-mounted sensors are available, but typically ceiling-mounted sensors give better coverage.

Figure 3.7   Wired motion wall sensor (Reproduced by permission of ABB)

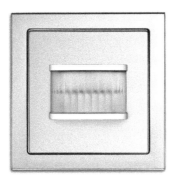

3.7 Photocells or brightness sensors

Traditional photocells switch loads on and off at a threshold of ambient brightness. A photocell that is analogue and connected to a smart home system can do much more – able, for example, to control shades to optimize lighting, lowering them to eliminate glare or raising them to 'harvest' natural light. Many smart home manufacturers supply a brightness sensor within a motion sensor module. This can be an efficient solution, but your design should consider the needs of the particular installation and you must be prepared to specify motion and brightness detection separately.

Figure 3.8 shows an integrated motion and brightness sensor on the left. On the right is an example of a compact sensor next to the dedicated module to which it must be connected in order to interpret its signal.

Figure 3.8   Brightness sensing devices (Reproduced by permission of Theben)

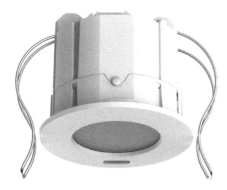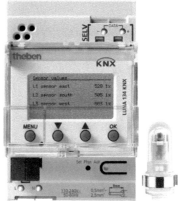

3.8 Door/window open/closed sensors

Historically associated with intruder alarms, these devices can also inform heating programmes or be used as an event trigger for any automation sequence. They should be installed at all designated openings, preferably on the opposite side to the hinge to guarantee sufficient clearance to trigger.

Figure 3.9   Door/window sensors (Reproduced by permission of Scolmore)

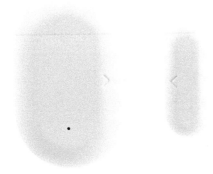

3.9 Wall button

Apps may be attractive, but some people still prefer a button (particularly if they can't find their phone). A button positioned on a wall or any other surface can therefore be set up to do anything that the system permits. Do note that retractive buttons are more common than rocker switches in smart homes: this is because the state of any part of the system should be determined by the central processor and not by the position of any given switch.

A typical smart home configuration would include one wall button per room, with large rooms and open-plan houses varying this requirement.

Figure 3.10   Wireless (left) and wired (right) buttons (Reproduced by permission of Ubiquiti Networks)

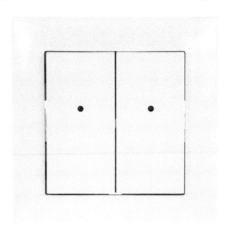 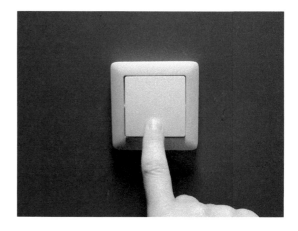

3.10 Temperature sensor

Smart heating is one of the main applications that have brought smart home technology and ideas into the mainstream.

Being able to control the heating of individual rooms offers improvements to economy and comfort. Analogue as opposed to digital (on/off thermostat) sensors give smart home heating systems another edge. A smart home climate control can balance itself based on temperature data and can show how heat moves around zones and out of the building. This can allow for weather compensation in the heating system – another requirement of Approved Document Part L: *Conservation of fuel and power* of the Building Regulations.

Typically, you should wire for one temperature sensor per room, with large rooms and open-plan houses varying this requirement. Smart temperature sensors still cannot tell if they have been installed above a radiator or inside a north-facing wall, so the usual rules regarding positioning continue to apply.

Figure 3.11   Wired (left) and wireless (right) temperature sensors (Reproduced by permission of Loxone and Ubiquiti Networks)

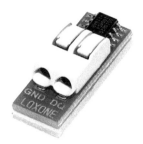
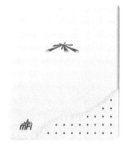

3.11 Thermal actuator

A thermal actuator is a device that controls flow through a radiator or an underfloor heating (UFH) manifold. It is also called a valve actuator (VA). In a smart home, a thermal actuator will have wired or wireless control via the UI. Many wireless VAs will have an inbuilt temperature sensor.

Note the following points about different types of VA:

(a) adaptors may be needed to match VAs to specific valves;
(b) VAs can be controlled by 230 V AC or DC (usually 24 V); and
(c) 24 V DC VAs can be digital (open/shut) or analogue (proportional opening, usually 0–10 V).

Figure 3.12   A valve actuator (Reproduced by permission of Theben)

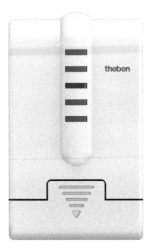

3.12 Shading: blind, shutter or curtain controllers

Blind, shutter or curtain controllers come in all shapes and sizes and can be wired or wireless. Some shades are battery-powered and controlled wirelessly. Wired shades may be 230 V AC or 24 V DC. Note that fitting particulars can vary between manufacturers and models.

Wiring to an outlet plate near the top, either side of the window, is standard practice. If specific shades have been specified, you might choose to bring the cable out unobtrusively, precisely where it is needed.

Figure 3.13 shows two possible forms of shading actuator. On the left is a DIN-mounted module that would sit in the HE and control multiple shades. On the right is a single controller that would be local to the shades and controlled from the HE.

Figure 3.13   Shading actuators (Reproduced by permission of Theben)

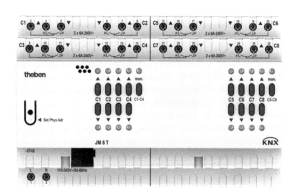

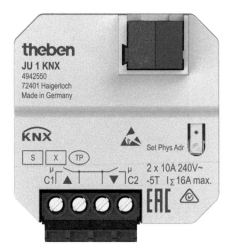

3.13 Fire detection

The installation of smoke alarms, or automatic fire detection systems, remains an important part of any home, as these increase the levels of safety by automatically giving an early warning of fire.

Many manufacturers offer smart solutions for smoke, heat and carbon monoxide alarms; however, it is important that you as the installer satisfy yourself of the requirements of Approved Document B Volume 1: *Dwellings* (ADB1) of the Building Regulations, which requires all new dwelling houses to be fitted with fire detection and fire alarm systems in accordance with BS 5839-6:2019 *Fire detection and fire alarm systems for buildings. Code of Practice for the design, installation, commissioning and maintenance of fire detection and fire alarm systems in domestic premises.* It is also worth bearing in mind that ADB1 stipulates specific product standards. These alarms should be checked against the manufacturer's data sheet of your chosen smart solution, as they may not comply.

Interestingly, any temperature sensor in a system can become a fire detector, in the same way as a kitchen heat detector is, by sensing a rapid rise in temperature and raising the alarm.

A smart home system might be linked to a traditional fire detection system through a simple contact closure, depending on design and manufacturers' guidelines.

Figure 3.14   A smart fire detector (Reproduced by permission of Loxone)

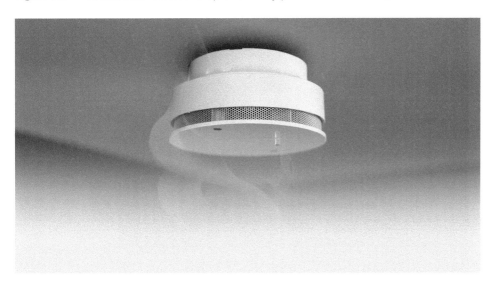

3.14 Security and access equipment

In smart homes there is often an overlap between lifestyle solutions and those areas that are fundamental for protecting lives, property and assets.

Security is as essential as ever; when discussing smart solutions, there is a need to be mindful of potential security hazards to ensure that these do not compromise overall physical security (or your customers' insurance policies). Security hazards need to be risk-assessed accordingly, with an appropriate grade of system installed. Where your system design affects access, you should always advise the client to check how it affects their insurance cover.

Many smart security measures feature remote monitoring, with the ability to activate alarms and automatically send signals, video and messages to mobile devices. It is worth knowing that these solutions will not result in police attendance unless there are additional indications from a person at the scene whilst a criminal offence is in progress. To achieve a police response, the intruder alarm system must hold a unique reference number (URN) and be installed, monitored and maintained by a company accredited by the United Kingdom Accreditation Service (UKAS) and an alarm receiving centre (ARC).

Most automated gates have a contact closure input, which can trigger them just as a pocket fob would. A smart home system can interface with this. Smart locks, however, are more controversial. Many people are not comfortable with the idea that someone could open their door by hacking into the security system that operates it. For those considering installing a smart lock in their property, one controlled door coupled with video surveillance or an intercom is perhaps a good safeguarding move.

Figure 3.15 shows one version of this concept: a lock/handle module paired with an app on a mobile device. There are many other versions, each of which has its own requirements. It is particularly important to refer to manufacturers' guidance when specifying access control.

Figure 3.15   App-controlled smart lock

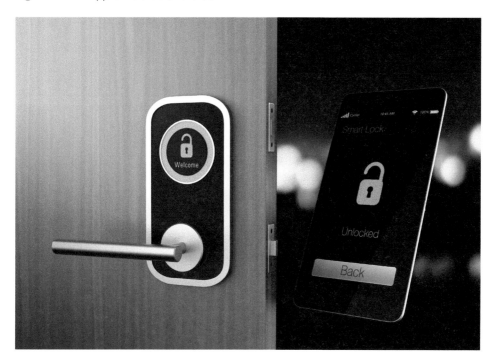

3.15 Energy-monitoring equipment

The UK government has mandated energy suppliers to upgrade every electricity and gas meter in the UK to a smart meter. The core function of a smart meter is to measure the energy in or out of a given building.

Good smart home design should incorporate infrastructure that will allow metering data to be used to manage energy, alongside the smart meter's capabilities, on the consumer's side.

Figure 3.16 shows two types of current-measuring equipment. On the left is a current transformer (CT) meter that is clamped round a cable so that it can measure current – this one has an RJ45 socket to allow for data to be extracted through an Ethernet cable. On the right is a DIN-mounted module that would be placed in-line at the origin of the circuit.

Figure 3.16   Cable clamp (left) and DIN-mounted energy meters (right) (Reproduced by permission of Ubiquiti Networks and Loxone)

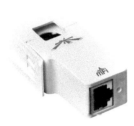
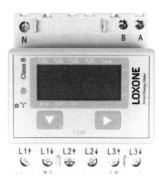

The resolution in which householders will want this kind of information will vary, according to factors including:

(a) the current-consuming equipment they have on-site;

(b) the microgeneration they have on-site;

(c) how much they care about saving energy;

(d) the availability of tariffs that reward energy management; and

(e) the cost-effectiveness of smart measures to provide data.

This application within smart homes is changing very quickly. The watchword here is 'future-ready' and the best advice is to get Ethernet cable to or near to all points where significant energy is likely to pass. These include:

(a) EV charge points;

(b) microgeneration at the inverter or point of grid connection;

(c) electrical heaters and high-wattage heating, ventilation and air-conditioning (HVAC devices) such as heat pumps;

(d) likely battery energy storage locations; and

(e) utility meters.

Note: Metering equipment and its accuracy are required to be matched to the application. Installers should consult manufacturers to ensure that any meters they install comply with relevant standards and regulations.

Figure 3.17 illustrates equipment that should be considered for consumption-monitoring when designing a smart home. Providing an Ethernet cable from the HE is one strategy for enabling energy-monitoring, but manufacturers' advice should be sought where possible to establish where additional physical and software interfaces may be required.

Figure 3.17   Equipment for which metering may be considered

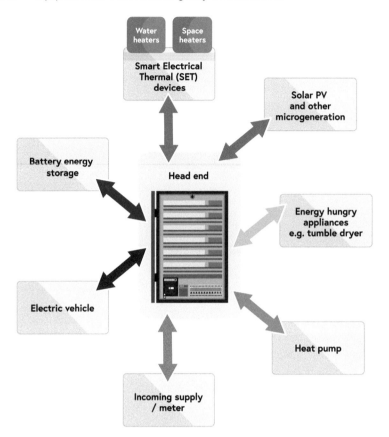

3.16 Audiovisual (AV) equipment

AV systems are a specialism in their own right. Many existing smart home specialists have historically been AV specialists happy to pick up the extra work with clients who have larger budgets.

For the electrical installer coming to this from the opposite direction, a note of caution is probably appropriate – and that is that designing and delivering high-end AV systems is tricky.

As an entrant, if the client wants the very best and latest AV system, the installer should consider teaming up with a specialist and coming to an understanding as to what cables they need you to install. The specialist can then concentrate on their own area of expertise.

It is possible to complete courses to gain proficiency in this area: see Appendix C for further information. Some products, aimed at the intermediate installer, are more manageable and have support offered. Some consumer-tech products plug and play directly with an internet connection – if the client is happy with these, and you have carried out your structured cabling properly, then the task will be successfully completed.

3.17 Summary

This Section has noted a range of equipment that a smart home installer might need to specify. Some categories have been very specific (for example, covering 'motion sensors'), whereas others have been more generic (for example, focusing on 'energy-monitoring equipment'). This reflects the fact that there are multiple ways to do many of the things needed in a smart home – and that smart home technology moves fast. Section 4 will now explore how to assess the client's smart home needs and then design to match those needs, rather than specifying from an outdated list.

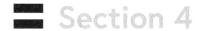

Capturing the client's requirements

This Section provides resources to help you create a conversation about what your client needs. The resources are templates that can be used as a project progresses, saving time and making it easier to secure good outcomes. There is also guidance on how to survey for a smart home job.

4.1   Back to the drawing board with the client

Standard electrical installation benefits from a luxury that is often taken for granted: it is mature technology, known and readily understood. A householder knows what a switch is, knows where it goes and knows what it does (it turns something on and off, usually nearby). The same is true for socket-outlets: these go where you need to plug things in. It is a tried and trusted template that traditional installation leans on heavily, and a crutch that allows us to skip a lot of electrical installer to householder communication.

With a smart home, that crutch disappears. Few clients will have a strong understanding of the products and their possibilities and those that do will need to explain their vision, which might be different to yours. An electrical installer must take a step back and remove the assumptions that come with traditional electrical installation.

Figure 4.1 illustrates how differently a client and designer may visualize a finished smart home. There may, for example, be agreement that solar power and energy management is good – but a difference in what each considers acceptable to be visible on the roof.

Figure 4.1   Client's vision of their smart home versus the designer's vision

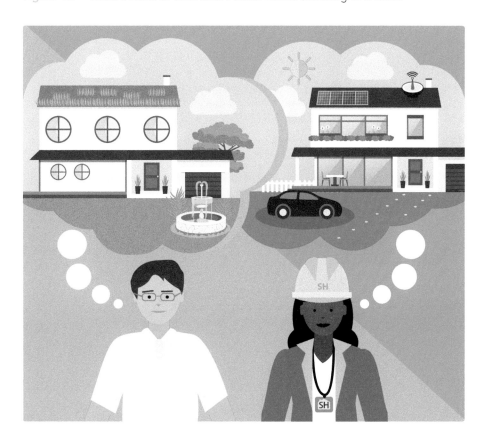

4.2 The needs analysis

A needs analysis is simply an analysis of the needs of the client. It provides a way of capturing the client's vision and breaking it down into deliverable parts, setting out expectations and confirming exactly what needs to be achieved.

It is important that clients create their own needs list.

This process might begin before a site visit or meeting with a phone or email conversation. Carrying out an in-depth survey, design and specification for every contact is unlikely to be sustainable – a preliminary needs analysis might be enough to establish that this job is not for you.

Assuming this is not the case and you take the job on, you should consider keeping better records of what is said than would normally be the case, while you become accustomed to the new possibilities.

4.2.1 Early contact

Appendix D provides a template designed for use on first contact. Whether this first contact is written or verbal, this template will help you to start documenting.

You will see familiar basics and some elements that might surprise you. For example, you might not be accustomed to asking potential clients how much time they spend in the house or who will be living in it – but that is the kind of information you need to do a good job. Done sensitively, this can also communicate to a client that you are able to see what they need and to deliver it.

4.2.2 Early contact documentation

An example of an early contact form is provided in Figure 4.2. This could be supplemented with other resources, such as images from Google Maps Street View, or plans as supplied by the client.

Figure 4.2   Smart home early contact template example

Name:

Jenny Trott

Client address:

New Barn, Station Road, Oldtown

Installation address:

Same as client

Starting when: March 20xx

Deadline for finish:

December 23rd 20xx

New build, rewire or retrofit measure:

New build (demolishing and rebuilding)

Size of installation:

5-bed home

Material: brick/block, timber frame, other:

Block and green oak frame.

Additional features on the property for connection:

Stable block, swimming pool and gate.

Questions to ask the client:

How would you describe the character of the finished installation?

Old-fashioned, but slick and stylish too.

When will people be there?

When working: all day every day, including early and late in the day and at weekends. Jenny works long hours out of the house, but her husband Carl is home all day when not travelling – which he does a lot. The couple go on holiday frequently.

Do you work from home?

The couple plan to have an office room which Carl will use. This needs to be locked most of the time, as Carl's employers insist on tight security.

What sort of functions or systems do you envisage in your smart home?

Jenny would like to be able to buzz people in when they come to the gate. Having beautiful lights is a big priority for the house – and also the garden, particularly if Jenny wants to go out for a swim in the evening when Carl is away, to feel a bit safer.

Who will be living in the home? Does anybody have any special needs?

Carl's father will be coming to live with them. They were going to build a separate cabin, the planned 'stable block', but he is getting a bit frail now, so they are thinking he might need to come into the house with them instead. However, they are not certain of this and he might have to go somewhere with specialist care.

What sort of things do you enjoy doing at home?

The couple enjoy listening to music and drinking cocktails. Carl likes to cook and also plans to spend time in his wood workshop, where he is making a boat. He might want a detached workshop-garage.

Is there anything I haven't asked about that you'd like me to consider?

The east side of the building is going to be entirely made of glass.

The couple might sell and move to Australia next year.

Notes:

Are there actually any horses?

Where is the swimming pool: is it in another building or outside?

4.2.3 Early contact analysis

'Jenny' is a fictitious character, but entirely within parameters for a smart home client. There is a great deal of information contained within this template (note the deadline, to start with)!

The colour coding in the template is designed to indicate how the communication might deviate from the traditional map. Blue shows where the conversation starts to veer away from the standard; yellow indicates where Jenny is being receptive to questions and offering information beyond what is strictly being asked; and green marks the point where Jenny is fully engaged and is indirectly telling you things that you really need to know in order to design her smart home.

It is important to stress that you might choose to omit or defer questions depending on how the quality of the contact unfolds. Getting to the end of your questions won't help with design if the client feels invaded. Similarly, if you simply received a call to see if you could fit their Nest thermostat the following week, those questions might seem a bit much.

As an exercise, let's pick out some things you have learned from that template that might have a bearing on smart home design:

(a) there are an unconfirmed number of features outside of the main house that might need to be included in the design.
(b) the client's 'old fashioned, but slick and stylish too' aesthetic ideal is not straightforward.

(c) the couple have quite a hectic lifestyle and are away a lot.

(d) there is a home-office requirement.

(e) there is likely to be a heightened requirement for cyber security, given what we have learned about Carl's work.

(f) the lighting requirement is a priority for Jenny.

(g) feeling safe and secure is a priority for Jenny: she wants gate entry and good lighting on the grounds.

(h) there is a possibility that one occupant might have a requirement for assisted living measures. If they do, it's possible that this will be temporary, so any measures in this regard need also to be temporary, particularly if a sale the following year goes ahead.

(i) there are a lot of implications of the east side being made of glass, including for lighting, climate control and shading.

This list of inferences is by no means exhaustive, but it gives you a real advantage for the next stage of communication. Thus armed, you can be the electrical installer who gets back to the client to offer considerations and suggestions that are relevant to them, and which they have perhaps not even considered yet themselves. Some examples might include the following:

(a) you might ask the client for some visual examples of the look they desire. Be prepared to use Pinterest or Instagram if they do. These can be very powerful consultation tools, not least because they operate remotely, saving you time and resources.

(b) a security system was not requested, but is strongly suggested by the gate and by Jenny's comments about how she feels when Carl is away. Jenny has told us that she is safety-conscious, so has she thought about how living under glass in the evening might feel on dark nights? Will automated shading be required?

(c) smart homes work well for people who are away a lot. Functional systems that have not been requested but that you might promote in this context include:

   (i) automated heating to save money and to allow for a comfortable temperature when they walk through the door;

   (ii) presence simulation;

   (iii) subject to the rules signposted in Section 3.14, smart systems can enable remote surveillance in addition to standard intruder detection for monitoring and peace of mind; and

   (iv) many systems allow an 'away mode', which automates all of the above items and more at the touch of a button, from anywhere with a data signal.

An automated heating system was not mentioned on the template, but will almost certainly be required. At an appropriate point, some questions you might ask about this include:

(a) has Jenny thought about how the glass east wall will affect the temperature? This room will get a lot of morning sun, which is another reason to suggest shading for the hotter months, and to keep in heat in the darker, colder months. Is contingency for air-conditioning also advisable?

(b) will there be any renewable systems, such as solar thermal, PV or heat pumps? The answers on the template would suggest that the client has the room and the budget for them.

Smart home infrastructure can lend itself very well to assisted living for Carl's father. Have the couple thought about how that might work to their advantage? See Appendix C for some resources that might be of benefit and share these with the client as appropriate.

A ten-minute conversation and ten minutes of note-taking could be all that is needed to build a good relationship with the client, which will help you to best match their needs.

More work is then required to take this information forward through the survey, design and delivery, and the Sections below will help you with this.

4.2.4 Consolidating the needs analysis

Communication in early contact is a very important aspect, and in the previous example, it was highly fruitful. A smart home project might involve unfamiliar technology, multiple construction phases and a large number of other trades and professions. It might also be worth significantly more than the projects to which you are accustomed. It is therefore a good idea to have a system in place for consolidating this general information.

After the early contact, there are key points you should aim to capture. Appendix D provides a template for consolidating needs. This is designed to help you keep your client's 'needs' within realistic boundaries, both for them and for your business.

Figure 4.3   Example of a consolidating needs template

This is a hypothetical consolidating needs scenario for a different client (Tom and Barbara). As with the early contact form, there is more information here than that which is explicitly written down.

Who is responsible for design?

The client has made drawings and has handed them over to an architect for optimization.

Are plans available?

The clients' drawings are available; the architects' drawings are pending.

Who is responsible for project management? A builder?

The client plans to project-manage hand-picked sub-contractors.

List of non-portable electrical equipment to be connected:

- EV charge point
- PV array
- battery energy storage
- hot water thermal store
- air source heat pump
- mechanical ventilation heat recovery (MVHR)
- dishwasher
- tumble-dryer
- freezer
- fridge
- wine fridge
- pond water fountain

List of systems the client would like to control:

- heating
- lighting
- garden irrigation

List of things the client would like to be able to monitor:

- plants in the greenhouse
- who comes to the door
- how much energy they use
- how much energy they send back to the grid

Figure 4.3   Cont

List of rooms by name, with a summary of their use and an indication as to whether they might change use:

- Living room – watching TV and reading books
- Dining room – eating and jigsaws
- Kitchen – cooking
- Utility room: laundry and heating equipment
- Hall – passing through
- Porch – storage for coats, hats and shoes
- Landing – passing through and also an exercise machine, maybe a cross-trainer
- Bed 1 – sleeping and yoga
- Bed 2 – sleeping
- Bed 3 – study and guest bed
- Bed 4 - sleeping
- Attic – storage and PV inverter
- Garage – car, tools and bikes

List of people who will occupy the home, including people who visit, e.g. cleaners/mobility team, children/grandchildren, parents/grandparents, pets:

Tom (Mr)

Barbara (Mrs)

Peter (child)

Jane (child)

Friends and family visit all the time. They will use the Bed 3 study, with a sofa bed in the living room as an overflow.

A cleaner comes once a week.

Pattern of occupancy, daily, seasonally:

Tom and Barbara own a business together and can be flexible about who goes to the office at any point. Either can work from home, which is why Bed 3 is a study. They would also like to be able to work downstairs when required. The children are at school and are old enough to come and go by themselves.

Does anyone in the home have any special needs?

No.

Does anyone work from home?

See above.

Is any later development planned?

Maybe a garden office chalet to cope with social overflow and for general enjoyment.

Are there any events or circumstances that should be anticipated?

Lots of parties: 60 or 70 people not unusual.

Is a change of occupancy or change of use likely?

Not for at least five years, until the children have left.

The garden office might become a yoga centre if Barbara completes her yoga training and they sell the business.

What is the budget for the project? What is the budget for electrics?

£1.2million/£25,000.

Any other information that might affect the requirements of the house:

Tom and Barbara want the house to be built out of straw bales.

The advantages of this exercise include the following:

(a) it provides a chance to gather information about plans and project management:
    (i) Tom is project-managing sub-contractors who do not regularly work together!
(b) a checklist of items and functional systems can be cross-referenced to identify gaps and overlaps:
    (i) the living room will actually be a bedroom when guests stay.
(c) you need to be able to design a list of anticipated devices and systems for control and monitoring:
    (i) there are major energy management requirements, including the greenhouse.
(d) the other questions can help to build a picture of how the householders will live in the house, now and in the future:
    (i) considering the possibility of big parties in a straw bale house, it might be an idea to increase the specification of the fire detection system!

4.3 The functional analysis

Completed early contact and consolidating needs forms might well hold all the information realistically needed to design the smart home that the client needs. However, this information is not yet in a form that can be given to a builder or a technician and is certainly not suitable as a basis for an agreement or contract.

The next step is therefore to turn the needs analysis into something more concrete: a functional analysis.

The needs analysis is the basis of the functional analysis. The functional analysis explains in non-technical but quantifiable terms how the home will function.

To be fair to yourself and to the client, the functional analysis should favour features and functions that can realistically be matched to available equipment and the client's budget.

Specific technical requirements need not be finalized in the functional analysis. At this point, everything could be represented in a diagram as a simple shape or symbol.

Templates for functional analysis can be found in Appendix D.

The extent of the functional analysis will reflect the extent of the householder's requirement. A short-form functional analysis template is included in Appendix D for stand-alone applications.

For a stand-alone WiFi camera, this might be completed as in Figure 4.4.

Figure 4.4 Example of a short-form functional analysis

Short-form functional analysis

Client:

Install date:

Zone/Room:
External wall of garage

Function:
X1 WiFi camera to be supplied by client, powered by existing plug inside garage. Cable from product plug to camera to be trunked. WiFi connection to come from the home router, which the client has checked is suitable.

Notes:

It is likely that you have prepared many estimates which look just like that – and indeed, you may well have carried out a job just like this.

Figure 4.5 gives an example of a functional analysis for a multi-featured smart home.

Figure 4.5   Example of a multi-zone functional analysis

Multi-zone functional analysis:

Zone/Room:

Living room

Function:

- 8 downlights, dimmable, controlled by physical switch in room, also by the system through the UI.

- X1 LED strip, colour changing and dimmable, to be concealed in coving around the wall close to the ceiling, pointing upwards to light the ceiling. Controlled by a physical switch in the room, also by the system through the UI.

- X3 outlets to control table lamps. Controlled by a physical switch in the room, also by the system through the UI.

- Thermal actuators (number to be confirmed) to control underfloor heating loops in the room – location of manifold to be confirmed.

- Temperature sensor linked to system – location to be confirmed.

- Motion sensor linked to system – location to be confirmed. This should be able to trigger lighting if that is desired (to be confirmed).

- X1 switch by the door to control lighting and blinds.

- X2 blind controllers to operate blinds to be sourced by client. Controlled by physical switch in room, also by the system through the UI.

- X2 Ethernet outlets behind the TV and music centre location.*

- X2 RG6 coaxial outlets behind the TV location.*

- X1 WiFi access point on the ceiling.

- X4 speaker cables to ceiling.*

- *Audiovisual equipment to be installed by others. Client will instruct AV installers to liaise to confirm spec of 1st fix and space requirements.

- 13 A socket-outlets – number and location to be confirmed.

Zone/Room:

Plant room (location to be confirmed)

Function:

Cabinet(s) to house devices necessary to provide automation and connectivity to the specification agreed in the functional analysis.

This is quite a jump from the WiFi camera. Points to notice include the following:

(a) there are now unconfirmed details and requirements (several 'to be confirmed's);
(b) there are now other trades and professions involved, who you will have to allow time to communicate with, including IT/network designers, AV specialists, shading installers and builders responsible for the light-emitting diode (LED) coving; and
(c) the only 'standard' item left, the 13 A socket-outlets, is still included.

Some established smart home installers ask for a fee for consultation beyond early contact. Beginners may not feel inclined to charge for consultation, but should nevertheless protect themselves and the householder from the consequences of misunderstandings by providing a functional analysis. An electrical installer should not begin to design the system until a functional analysis has been completed and signed off as agreed.

Another equally compelling reason to complete a functional analysis is that, if done correctly, it can save you time and effort down the line. This makes for a better and more profitable project.

4.4 The survey

Universal survey items include, but are not limited to:

(a) site access assessment;
(b) site safety assessment;
(c) environment assessment; and
(d) an overview of existing electrical installation.

A survey may not be necessary for straightforward jobs. As an electrical installer, you may have products and services you offer on a speculative price basis without survey and find that this works well for you. Familiarity with the product is the key to this strategy.

Where the environment is existing, and not off-plan, it is recommended that you perform a survey for smart home work.

Remember that virtual resources like Google's satellite and Street View can provide a good understanding of the scale and aspect of the client's home without an on-site visit.

It might be advisable to conduct a phased survey, beginning with a general one while you are establishing viability and interest. Following this, you might return to survey in more detail, for example, carrying out:

(a) an itemization of rooms with elevation diagrams;
(b) a detailed survey of existing 'legacy' cabling; and
(c) heat mapping (of connectivity; see Section 4.4.1) by agreement, if required.

4.4.1 Smart home survey factors

Factors that might need extra consideration include:

(a) building fabric;
(b) electromagnetic compatibility (EMC);
(c) connectivity;
(d) grid stability; and
(e) inflation of processes and materials.

Figure 4.6   Example of building fabric that can cause interference

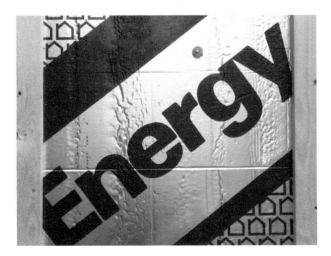

Materials that can block wireless and WiFi are considered in more detail in Section 6.

Figure 4.7   Some devices which can cause interference and issues with EMC

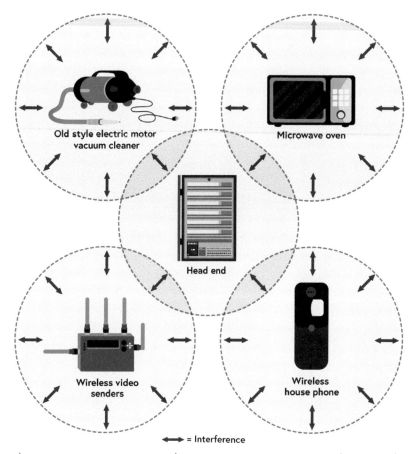

Issues that can stop equipment working or communicating properly are explored in Section 5.

Connectivity

Is internet connectivity good? If remote functionality is required, could this be a weak link?

Mobile data strength might be an issue if a device uses a SIM (subscriber identification module) card or communicates via SMS (short messaging service). It could be a significant factor when you need technical support onsite from a manufacturer.

Wired internet speed can be established using an online speed checker. However, the reliability of this needs to be established.

An indication of WiFi or mobile signal might be gained by moving around with devices and looking at the 'bars' on the display; however, this method is not considered to be reliable. Apps can be loaded onto smart devices to better analyse signal data – and these can improve understanding, albeit only a little.

Figure 4.8   Examples of mobile and PC apps to analyse signal data

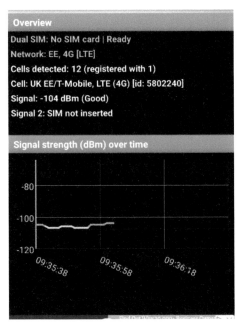

Dedicated equipment can be bought to analyse all bands of mobile signal, but not all produce reports, which might be needed.

Figure 4.9   Hand-held signal analyzer (Reproduced by permission of RF Explorer Technologies)

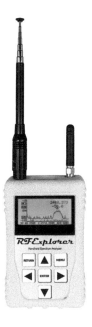

If the needs analysis indicates that connectivity-resilience is a critical concern, consider suggesting that a specialist carries out 'heat mapping' of WiFi, internet connection and mobile signal strength as appropriate. This is a specialist field requiring expensive equipment. Practitioners should produce a report that can be used for design and even sent to manufacturers for confirmation that their equipment will work in a given location.

This measure can improve outcomes. In the worst-case scenario, it can limit your liability if things do not work as hoped.

Grid stability

Rural locations are more vulnerable to power outages and transient voltages. Voltage spikes and lightning strikes can be extremely expensive and disruptive in a smart home.

Regulation 443.4 of the IET Wiring Regulations (BS 7671:2018+A1:2020) states:

> *Protection against switching overvoltages shall be considered in the case of equipment likely to produce switching overvoltages or disturbances exceeding the values according to the overvoltage category of the installation.*

A reasonably well featured smart home is likely to be worth the installation of protective measures by the installer and/or enhanced insurance by the client.

Guidance on the selection and installation of appropriate surge protection devices (SPDs) can be found in Section 534 of BS 7671:2018+A1:2020. It is worth noting that Ethernet over Power (EOP) and PLC signals may not pass through protective devices such as residual current devices (RCDs). Installers should check manufacturers' data to ensure compatibility.

Inflation of processes and materials

When conducting a smart home site analysis, keep in mind that processes and materials may be more extensive than usual.

Examples of this include the following concerns:

(a) assembling the HE of a fully-featured smart home can take days: could this upset the plans of the electrical installer or other people?
(b) the volume of the cables back to the HE might come as a surprise. Is there room to route them properly?
(c) is there room for the enclosures that are required?
(d) has allowance been made for additional travel time, accommodation, etc.?

4.5   Project documents

4.5.1   Why documentation is important

In a smart home project, staying on track with documentation is vital:

(a) to manage the increased demands of complicated and unfamiliar elements; and
(b) to facilitate the handover of a complete 'user manual' for the householder.

Figure 4.10   Possible elements of a handover pack

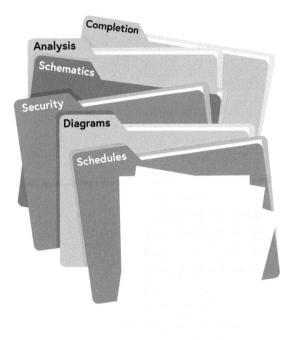

4.5.2 Documentation up to this point

By now, at least three very important documents (dealt with in Sections 4.2–4.4) should have been created:

1. Needs analysis

(a) The early contact form: an opportunity to capture basics and the householder's vision of what they want.
(b) The consolidating needs form: an opportunity to get more detail of how the project will proceed. Provides lists of requirements that can be cross-checked to improve understanding and identify the questions that need to be asked.

2. The site survey

If carried out. If the building is off-plan, you should have a copy of that plan.

3. Functional analysis

A non-technical document that describes the functionality that it should be possible to demonstrate at the end of the job.

4.5.3 The many uses of the functional analysis

The needs analysis documents might never surface again, but, if done properly, the functional analysis will serve as the basis for:

(a) all design documents;

(b) a brief for a manufacturer or supplier and useful reference if the products they supply do not fit the requirement;

(c) your estimate;

(d) the basis for a contract or agreement, if included with a proposal;

(e) a reference in meetings on- and off-site, useful in challenging scope creep and misunderstandings; and

(f) the commissioning checklist at handover.

4.6 Summary

This Section has offered a framework to structure your consultation and documentation in the early stages of a project.

Remember that each client will be different. An electrical installer may well have a client who is a developer, reselling afterwards. It is most likely that all they will want is an assured margin – and they will expect the electrical installer to have the answers.

For householders:

(a) from the outset, don't assume that the clients have been informed of the possibilities;

(b) remember that many clients won't know what can be achieved;

(c) take care to inform the client – make the technology accessible;

(d) always explain within the context of their requirements; and

(e) always explain the benefit, not the technology.

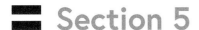 Section 5

Safety aspects of smart home design

This Section flags up some of the ways in which ensuring health and safety with a smart home, both during and after installation, might require extra attention compared with a standard installation.

5.1 The standard for safety

The UK construction industry takes its lead on safety in projects from the Construction (Design and Management) Regulations 2015 (CDM).

The CDM Regulations place obligations on all the parties involved in construction projects, including domestic projects, where there is more than one contractor.

The central roles are:

(a) the client – the party who orders the work to be done;
(b) the principal contractor (PC) – the party responsible for carrying out the work; and
(c) the principal designer (PD) – the party responsible for the design of the work.

An electrical installer might find that they are the best candidate on a project for the PC or the PD role. A smart home installer is more likely than others to be the best candidate on a project, due to their increased involvement in design, installation, documentation and consultation. While that involvement might sound onerous, installers should bear in mind that in doing a good job and keeping good records, they will be fulfilling most CDM requirements anyway.

5.2 The smart home safety challenge

Regulation 134.1.1 of BS 7671:2018+A1:2020 refers to good workmanship by skilled or instructed persons and the use of proper materials in the erection of electrical installations. It also refers to the need to take account of manufacturers' instructions. Regulation 510.3 states:

> Every item of equipment shall be selected and erected so as to allow compliance with the regulations stated in this chapter and the relevant regulations in other parts of BS 7671 and shall take account of manufacturers' instructions.

As you enter the smart home industry, you will probably be working with systems with which you are less familiar. This means that more work is required to:

(a) deliver the systems as intended;
(b) ensure safety during the installation; and
(c) ensure the operational safety of the finished installation.

It is also possible that this type of work will lead into larger projects, which will require enhanced project and safety documentation.

When stepping into this new and more challenging role, you should take the opportunity to adopt a more comprehensive 'designing for safety' approach.

5.3 Designing for safety

Where materials and systems are unfamiliar, but the health and safety requirements are the same, you need to take steps to ensure that you are complying.

Consider, firstly, moving away from the stand-alone risk assessment. Aim instead to capture, identify and incorporate information that is relevant to safety as you progress through the job. For example:

(a) highlight operational safety considerations (things that might happen when the system is in use). These should be identified at the needs analysis stage and, where appropriate, referenced in the functional analysis. See Appendix D for an example template you might use.

(b) identify on-site hazards in your survey.

(c) where specifying unfamiliar equipment of reasonable complexity, it is a good idea to spend time on diagrams within a method statement. The diagrams and method statements will inform each other and help you to identify gaps before these affect the project. Discovering, for instance, that a previously unthought-of and unknown part is missing, and takes a week to arrive, can be problematic. See Appendix D for an example method statement template.

Appendix C provides signposts to resources to help you develop your practice with respect to safety and the CDM Regulations. It is recommended that you adopt the systems noted, as they offer an approach that can save you time and improve the safety and quality of the installation.

5.3.1 Operational safety

The designer must consider the safety of the system as-installed to the user. Standard electrical installation has very well-established do's and don'ts; Approved Document P: *Electrical Safety – Dwellings* of the Building Regulations, commonly referred to as 'Part P', took up the challenge of standardizing these to protect householders from un-informed and dangerous practices.

Standardization has not happened yet for smart homes specifically, but there are extra considerations that a designer must take into account where systems take on more monitoring and control.

Below, we consider some example situations.

Your client might ask you to automate a bed to fold up into the wall on a timer when they have gone to work. This is easily done – but what if someone else is still inside the bed?

You might be asked to design and programme for a system that relies entirely on web-based UIs. That will not be of any use if the home router breaks. This situation could also create hazards. Have you recommended some physical override switches for critical systems, such as heating, access and lighting?

Relying solely on WiFi or a wireless connection to control devices can be hazardous. A signal problem could result in a situation where it is not possible to turn lights on when they are needed for safety.

You might recommend a UPS to a client. Let's imagine that a smart home system has been installed as an assisted living measure for an elderly parent. A permitted family member might like to be notified of power cuts in that parent's house. You might install the hardware to do this and do the programming – but if the power cut disables both elements before the message goes out, that measure will fail.

Similarly, where wireless or battery-powered devices are used, there should be provision to ensure that batteries are maintained.

The new possibilities a smart home offers can create other problems. For example, a system might allow users to group lights together under a single 'on' command. If those lights have a combined inrush current that exceeds the protective device, the installation could suffer an outage.

Section 5 – Safety aspects of smart home design

If you take on work to design a system that is intended to address physical infirmities, your safety remit now legally extends beyond electrical safety into functional and operational safety and you have an obligation to identify and design for safety critical systems (SCSs). The operational safety template in Appendix D might be used towards this purpose, but the installer will have ultimate responsibility for due diligence.

Figure 5.1   Safety critical systems and functional safety scenarios

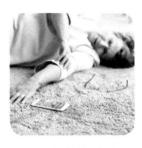 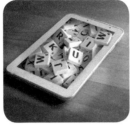 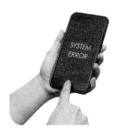

A person with a physical or mobility issue might be unable to access a control point if access is not planned for.

Conversely smartphone-based automation might enable someone with a disablity. A fallen resident or carer might be able to open a door to let paramedics in.

Automation can be an enabler for those with cognitive challenges or in some cases their carers.

There are many pitfalls however. Such a person might struggle to close the windows on a cold night if the user-interface is not well designed for purpose.

'Cognitive challenge' encompasses a huge spectrum. Each case and user should be considered unique. Mild dyslexia can be a barrier to inclusion if the UI is too 'texty'. In such a case, favour icon-based interfaces.

With vulnerable end-users in particular, safety goes beyond electrical safety to functional or operational safety.

Where you cannot guarantee the UI is infallible, provide physical back up controls with instructions for when the smart stuff fails.

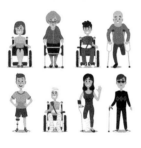 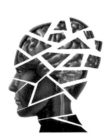 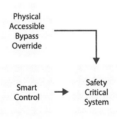

5.4   Smart home earthing and bonding

5.4.1   Scope and definitions

In Section 5.3 we considered how smart home system malfunctions might have serious consequences for householders and users. A smart home designer should therefore take extra steps to ensure that the equipment specified is not adversely affected by its environment. For example, systems that rely on electronic communication and processing can be adversely affected by EMI. To some extent, smart home manufacturers should design their products to have immunity from EMI, but this cannot be assumed. A smart home designer should therefore take steps to minimize the risk that EMI will impair the systems they install.

Section 5 – Safety aspects of smart home design

The design of low voltage (LV) earthing systems for automatic disconnection of supply (ADS), as listed in Table 5.1, is outside the scope of this Guide. This Guide will highlight practices that have been uncommon in domestic electrical installations, but which may be beneficial in smart homes.

To begin, we should review the definitions of three common forms of earthing connection.

Table 5.1   LV earthing definitions

Earthing: connection of the exposed-conductive-parts of an installation to the main earthing terminal (MET) of that installation, for example, the metal case of an electric heater.

Equipotential bonding: electrical connection maintaining various exposed-conductive-parts and extraneous-conductive-parts at substantially the same potential, for example, a metallic gas utility pipe that enters the property.

Functional earth: earthing of a point or points in a system or in an installation or in equipment, for purposes other than electrical safety, such as for the proper functioning of electrical equipment.

Table 5.2   EMI

Electromagnetic interference (EMI) is also known as 'coupling'.

The coupling can be via a conductive path, such as a wire or other metallic object (common impedance coupling), or at a distance through a medium such as air (capacitive, inductive or radiated coupling).

Coupling is typically described as being between a *source* and a *victim* or between a *disturber* and a *disturbed*.

The source can be another device, a cable or atmospheric conditions.

When coupling occurs, the energy of one system will disturb the energy of another system.

Coupling can cause malfunctions or destroy electronic equipment.

5.4.2 The requirement for measures to mitigate EMI

The most important step a smart home designer can take to mitigate EMI is to ensure that all equipment they install is EMC-approved for the intended environment.

Products intended for the European Market should bear the 'CE' mark that indicates EMC compliance and compliance with other relevant standards. It is recommended that UK smart homes should only contain electromechanical equipment that bears the CE mark.

In a house where:

(a) all electrical and electronic products are CE-marked and comply with appropriate standards and have satisfactory EMC performance; and
(b) all cabling and equipment has been installed as required by the relevant standards, including BS 7671:2018+A1:2020 and BS 6701:2016 *Telecommunications equipment and telecommunications cabling. Specification for installation, operation and maintenance*;

there should be no need for any special measures with respect to EMI.

Note: BS 7671:2018+A1:2020 requires BS 6701 also to be used for telecommunications installations.

Modern control cables (i.e. anything other than auxiliary contacts, current-loop and analogue voltage control) come under the definition of telecommunications in BS 6701. Home and building electronic systems (HBES)/smart homes equipment have wired or wireless networking or other data connectivity and may therefore be classed as telecommunications equipment.

5.4.3 Factors encouraging measures to mitigate EMI

A smart home designer cannot control all the factors involved with the installation or the environment occupied by the installation. Circumstances that might undermine the assumption outlined in Section 5.4.2 and create a requirement for special measures to mitigate EMI include:

(a) installation in an environment where others have done electrical or electronic installation that may not be compliant.

(b) installation in an environment containing other devices that may not be compliant.

(c) installation of devices that lack the CE mark.

(d) installation of devices that are faulty or counterfeit and may not comply with the accreditation they claim. This is to be avoided where possible, but it can happen.

Where there is a chance that the existing conditions, or future conditions, might create EMI, it is in the interests of all parties involved that a smart home designer takes reasonable precautions when designing.

5.4.4 An outline of measures to mitigate EMI

The remainder of this Section deals with three measures to mitigate the effects of EMI in smart homes:

1. earthing and bonding;
2. segregation (which also has implications for basic protection); and
3. shielding and screening.

Note: These are not the only safety issues to consider. Other technical areas specific to smart homes, for example, the provision of remote DC power and surge protection, will be dealt with in Sections 6–8.

In a smart home, all the measures prescribed for earthing and bonding in a standard installation, as required by BS 7671:2018+A1:2020, should be in place. The differences in earthing that might be implemented to better protect sensitive smart home equipment from EMI include the following:

(a) the protective (safety) earthing might be adapted; and

(b) bonding might be extended and enhanced to create functional earthing.

5.4.5 Adjustments to protective earthing and bonding conductors

We will first consider how the protective (safety) earthing might be adapted. Some basic measures, with familiar elements, that can reduce EMI include:

(a) securing the lowest possible earth fault loop impedance (Z_e) for the installation: TN systems (protective multiple earthing (PME) or TN-C-S and TN-S) distributor-provided earthing arrangements are almost always best, because they have the lowest impedance to earth.

(b) where a local TT earth connection is the only option, strive to achieve a connection that is ≤20.0 Ω. This may necessitate the use of a foundation earth electrode or other means superior to a standard earth rod. It may not be possible to achieve this in some installations.

(c) minimizing the length of the main earthing conductor (MEC) and other main protective bonding conductors will reduce the possibility that they will be subject to inductive coupling. Creating a centralized hub for all services near to building entrance facilities (BEFs) where possible will facilitate this. Where possible, try to keep the distance between the length of the MEC and the MET at ≤2.5 m.

Section 5 – Safety aspects of smart home design

5.4.6 Functional earthing and bonding

Considerations with regard to the extension and creation of functional earthing are far more extensive. To begin with, we shall outline the objectives of the exercise:

(a) to create a low impedance pathway to earth for all metallic objects in the structure, so that disturbing energy can be absorbed into the general mass of Earth before it can disturb electronic equipment.

(b) to create the most equipotential zone possible throughout the structure and the electromechanical devices within it. This includes metallic objects that are not extraneous. Materials such as metal in frame walls cannot be touched, but can interact with the electromagnetic energy of other systems at a distance.

Annex A444 of BS 7671:2018+A1:2020 (Measures Against Electromagnetic Disturbances) illustrates four formats for 'Structures for the network of bonding conductors and earthing conductors':

   1. protective conductors in a star network;
   2. a multiple meshed bonding star network;
   3. a common meshed bonding star network; and
   4. protective conductors connected to a bonding ring conductor.

The first is a layout shown below, which will be familiar to domestic electrical installers, as it is prevalent in standard domestic electrical installation. In the majority of smart home installations, where products and infrastructure are compliant as outlined in Section 5.4.2, this will be an adequate way to connect equipment to the MET.

Figure 5.2   Standard earthing arrangement

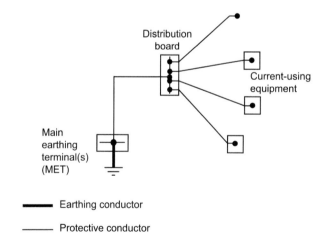

Examples 2–4 can be seen in Annex A444.1.2–1.4. All depict arrangements where equipment is connected to metallic structures within the building. A composite of these formats is shown in Figure 5.3.

Section 5 – Safety aspects of smart home design

Figure 5.3   Examples of equipotential bonding networks in a structure without a lightning protection system

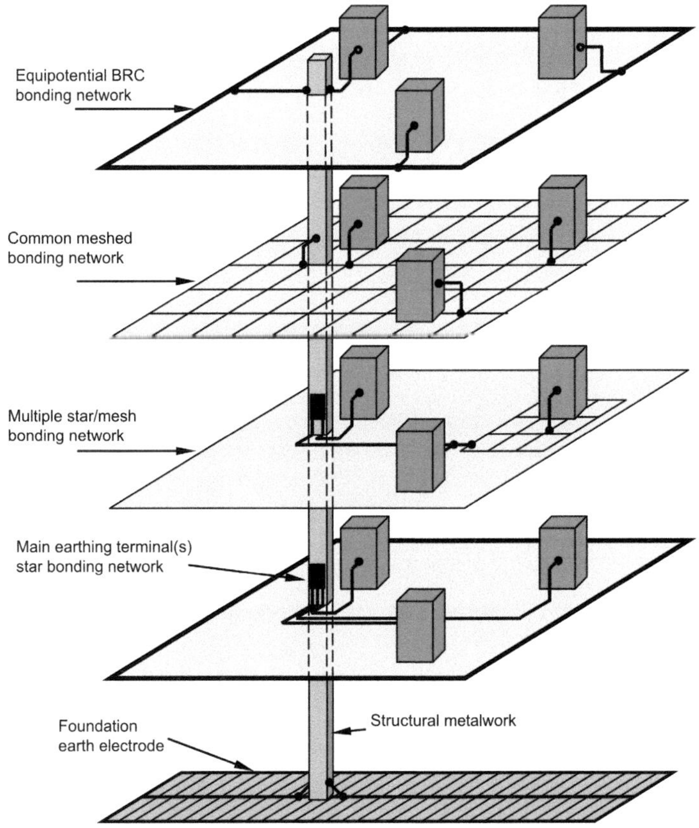

- Equipotential BRC bonding network
- Common meshed bonding network
- Multiple star/mesh bonding network
- Main earthing terminal(s) star bonding network
- Foundation earth electrode
- Structural metalwork

The connection formats in Figure 5.3 show how equipment-earth connections might be made more numerous where the density of electronic equipment is increased.

The goal of the strategies noted above is to reduce the earth fault loop impedance as far as possible by:

(a) creating parallel paths to earth; and
(b) increasing the surface area of the contact with earth.

Formats 2–4 are likely to far exceed the protective earthing requirements for compliance with BS 7671:2018+A1:2020 for a dwelling and as such may be described as functional earthing.

Of the four formats, the common meshed bonding star network is considered to be the most effective. However, in practice, a smart home designer would be very unlikely to adopt any of the formats as shown here in a smart home, because to do so would be expensive and unaesthetic.

The next Section will describe some measures that a smart home installer might implement to gain some of the potential benefits of the measures illustrated above, without excessive cost or aesthetic implications.

5.4.7 Functional earthing at the first fix stage

With a new-build or rewire project, the smart home designer has the opportunity to install functional earthing measures at low cost – a small fraction of the cost of remedial measures, should EMI prove to be an issue on commissioning. Measures to be considered include:

(a) adjustments to standard earthing and bonding conductors as described in Section 5.4.5.
(b) bonding conductor connections from the MET to significant non-extraneous metallic structures within the building (see Notes 1 and 2). Consider, in particular, those that:
    (i) have a connection to the general mass of Earth; or
    (ii) have a grid or mesh configuration that could create a barrier or a 'Faraday cage' zone within the installation.
(c) bonding conductor connections between bonded structures (see Note 3).

Notes:

1. Regulation 543.5.1 of BS 7671:2018+A1:2020 states that "where earthing for combined protective and functional purposes is required, the requirements for protective measures shall take precedence."
It is best practice to specify functional bonding conductors that satisfy the conditions of protective bonding conductors, as in fault conditions such as a lightning strike, they are likely to carry the same current as protective bonding conductors. In practice, therefore, functional earth bonding conductors need to be the same size, as they are required to bond extraneous structural steel.

2. Do not neglect the labelling of these conductors at the head end, as they may be more difficult to access and verify than connections to incoming services.

3. As for Note 1, specify conductors that match the performance of protective bonding conductors.

5.4.8 Summary of measures for functional earthing at first fix

---

IET Wiring Regulations (BS 7671:2018+A1:2020), Regulation 542.4.1:

"In every installation a main earthing terminal shall be provided to connect the following to the earthing conductor:

    (i) The circuit protective conductors
    (ii) The protective bonding conductors
    (iii) Functional earthing conductors (if required)
    (iv) Lightning protection system bonding conductor, if any (see Regulation 411.3.1.2)."

Functional earthing does not in any way replace protective earthing. Protective earthing, as required by appropriate regulations, including BS 7671:2018+A1:2020, should always be in place. Where the installation is existing, the compliance of the earthing should be verified prior to design and installation.

For the avoidance of doubt, functional earthing is a branch of the overall earthing system and should not be isolated from it.

Functional earthing that is not part of the structural earthing arrangements, but part of the specified system, should be specified in consultation with the manufacturers of the specified system. In practice, this will be where cables or conductors within cables have a functional earthing role. Strategies for collaboration with smart home manufacturers will be covered in Section 7. Some guidance on specifying cables to mitigate EMI is contained in Section 5.6.2.

Note: Where the functional earth is used for telecommunications equipment, the cable has to be continuously marked with the words TELECOMMS FUNCTIONAL EARTH in accordance with Clause 5.2.2.3 of BS 6701. Functional earth conductors are currently cream in colour, but are due to be designated to be pink after September 2020.

Remember that the best way to avoid EMI issues is to ensure that the system you specify is EMC-compliant and that it is not adjacent to equipment that is not EMC-compliant.

Formats 2–4 in Section 5.4.6 are illustrative, not prescriptive, for smart homes. A smart home should not require a great deal of functional earthing infrastructure. The suggested approach is simply to bond what you can while it is easy and economical to do so.

5.5 Smart home equipment segregation

5.5.1 Intended outcomes of segregation

BS 7671:2018+A1:2020 is concerned with cable segregation for two reasons:

1. primarily, due to the risk that Band 1 (extra-low voltage (ELV)) circuits might, in a fault, become connected to higher Band 2 (LV) voltages for which they were not designed. This can result in lethal effects, including touch voltages and fire.
2. secondarily, due to the risk of detrimental influence by EMI or coupling, as discussed below.

IET Wiring Regulations (BS 7671:2018+A1:2020), Regulation 444.6.1 (Segregation of circuits. General):

Cables that are used at voltage Band II (low voltage) and cables that are used at voltage Band I (extra-low voltage) which share the same cable management system or the same route, shall be installed according to the requirements of Regulations 528.1 and 528.2. Circuits of the same voltage band might also require segregation or separation.

Electrical safety and electromagnetic compatibility might produce different segregation or separation requirements. The design shall meet both requirements.

Note: Therefore, as is the case with functional earthing and bonding, where functional bonding should be compliant with protective bonding standards, segregation for EMC should also be compliant with standards for segregation for energy transfer by conductive contact.

5.5.2 The hierarchy of measures for segregation

When organizing the physical placement of systems (including cables and wires) that are of different energy bands or that have the potential for one to disturb the other, in order of preference, the designer should implement at least one of the following measures:

1. place distance between them;
2. place containment or barriers between them;
3. ensure that insulation is sufficient to prevent energy transfer by conductive contact.

5.5.3 Distancing

Clause A444.4 (Design guidelines for segregation of circuits) of BS 7671:2018+A1:2020 states:

Where the specification and/or intended application of the information technology cable is not available, then the cable separation distance between the power and information technology cables should be a minimum of 200 mm in free air.
This distance can be reduced if a screened power cable, a metallic barrier, or containment system is used as described in Table A444.1.

There is detailed information in Annex A444, which a designer should consult. In normal conditions and using the cables that will be described later, this extract of Table 444.1 of this Annex is a useful guide:

Table 5.3   Extract of Table A444.1 of BS 7671:2018+A1:2020

Containment applied to the mains power cabling		
No containment or open metallic containment A[1]	Perforated open metallic containment B[2]	Solid metallic containment C[3]
200 mm	150 mm	Note 4

Section 5 – Safety aspects of smart home design

Under certain defined conditions, BS EN 50174-2:2018 *Information technology. Cabling installation. Installation planning and practices inside buildings* (as referenced by BS 7671:2018+A1:2020) may permit the above separation requirements for EMC to be reduced, provided that all requirements for separation for safety are met.

5.5.4 Containment and barriers

In Table 5.3, we see that the permissible distance between Band 1 and Band 2 systems reduces when the Band 2 cabling is increasingly enclosed in a metallic cable management system (CMS), such as tray or trunking.

Mitigation of EMI by these methods requires that the containment should be continuously bonded to the MET, thereby performing a functional earthing role.

Cable tray inhibits the EMI of cables, but the protection depends on the positioning of the cables, as shown in Figure 5.4. Note that structural steel such as an I-beam can create similar protection if it is continuously bonded back to the MET.

Figure 5.4   Cables within tray

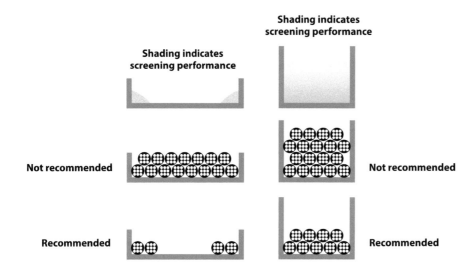

5.5.5 Smart home contingency segregation

Segregation by means of creating distance or incorporating barriers between different classes of equipment and cable can be more challenging in a smart home, due to the increased number of cables and circuit classes. Electrical installers will be aware that it is not always possible to implement the distances recommended above or to create bonded metallic containment within domestic installations, due to limitations of space. Designers and installers should use their own professional judgment in such circumstances to ensure that systems are safe as installed.

Contingencies include the use of:

(a) barriers such as flexible ducting.

(b) concentric steel-wired armour (SWA) for power cables. When bonded back to the MET, this will perform the same function as the solid metal containment listed in the extract from Table A444.1.

5.5.6 Insulation

This measure is concerned with conductive contact, rather than coupling.

Regulation 528.1 (Proximity of electrical services) of BS 7671:2018+A1:2020 lists measures that might make it possible to bring equipment of differing energy bands in close proximity to each another:

Except where one of the following methods is adopted, neither a voltage Band I nor a voltage Band II circuit shall be contained in the same wiring system as a circuit of nominal voltage exceeding that of low voltage, and a Band I circuit shall not be contained in the same wiring system as a Band II circuit:

(i)	Every cable or conductor is insulated for the highest voltage present
(ii)	Each conductor of a multicore cable is insulated for the highest voltage present in the cable
(iii)	The cables are insulated for their system voltage and installed in a separate compartment of a cable ducting or cable trunking system
(iv)	The cables are installed on a cable tray system where physical separation is provided by a partition
(v)	A separate conduit, trunking or ducting system is employed
(vi)	For a multicore cable, the cores of the Band I circuit are separated from the cores of the Band II circuit by an earthed metal screen of equivalent current-carrying capacity to that of the largest core of a Band II circuit.

Items (i)–(iii) outline requirements where distancing and barriers are not practical, and it has become necessary to have cables and conductors of different energy bands in close proximity to one another. This situation should be avoided wherever possible. Section 8 contains guidance on designing smart home HEs where this might be unavoidable.

Items (iv)–(v) outline how containment might be separated or partitioned to achieve segregation.

Item (vi) describes the criteria for the use of a cable to carry different energy bands. This compliance should be verified with the cable manufacturer and the smart home manufacturer.

5.6 Shielding and screening in smart home cables and equipment

5.6.1 Smart home equipment

Devices can be disruptors or disrupted by EMI without the presence of a cable. The needs analysis noted in Section 4.2 asked the client about the electrical devices to be connected. However, while your survey might have been thorough, modern electrical and electronic items can creep in unannounced and swamp delicately balanced signals. If a householder has a known EMI disruptor such as a welder, you should find out where such items will be and design away from them, as shown in outline in Figure 5.5.

Section 5 – Safety aspects of smart home design

Figure 5.5   Example of potential EMI disruption

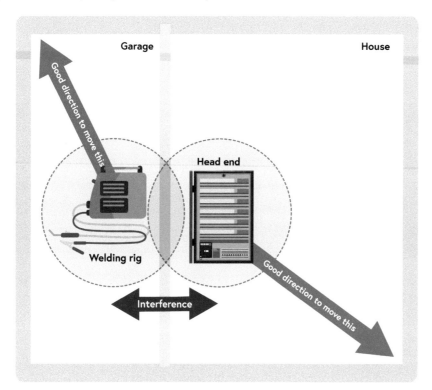

It is possible to have instruments that produce EMI but are EMC-compliant, because they have functionally earthed metallic casing that completely surrounds them.

Where there is no surrounding metallic casing, but levels of EMI are low enough, ferrite beads may be used. These are commonly found on switching power supplies. Ferrite beads on power leads for IT equipment are intended to inhibit EMI from devices if this might otherwise exceed levels permitted by EMC directives.

Figure 5.6   Ferrite bead on power lead

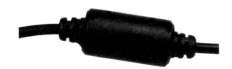

5.6.2   Smart home cables

Smart home equipment manufacturers should be able to guide the smart home designer as to which cables to use to connect their equipment.

Provision for smart home equipment that is an electrical load is covered in Section 6 of this Guide.

With respect to smart home cables, which we will term 'telecommunications' cables, equipment that requires signals will typically be served by the home's structured cabling. The majority of smart home structured cabling will be done with balanced and symmetrical cables, usually Category (CAT) CAT6A or above cables.

5.6.3 CAT cables

CAT cables are extremely versatile. Properties that make them reliable for communication include the following:

(a) they are symmetrical. Each pair is twisted to a precise degree throughout the length of the cable, which reduces the interference that would occur if they were run parallel.

(b) they are balanced. The resistance per metre is regulated to prevent reflections of impulses that can make the signal less coherent.

Note that copper-clad aluminium (CCA) 'network cable', whilst affordable, is not good enough for structured cabling infrastructure.

Figure 5.7 illustrates the structure of CAT cable, including the use of shielding, which is explained.

Figure 5.7   4-twisted pair CAT cable shielding

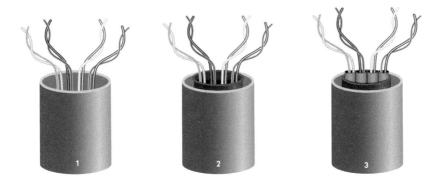

Figure 5.7 indicates the structure of three types of CAT cable.

1. In Example 1, there is a basic unscreened CAT cable. Lacking any concentric shielding, it is more susceptible to external EMI.

2. Example 2 shows a screened CAT cable that has a concentric metallic screen or braid surrounding the twisted pairs, but inside the external sheath. If that metallic sheath is connected to the MET, this would constitute a functional earth connection. This cable would therefore provide a greater degree of protection from external EMI than the cable in Example 1.

3. Example 3 shows an enhanced cable, with screening of the four sets of twisted pairs in addition to the outer screen or braid found in the second example. If all these screens are bonded to the MET, then this cable protects the signal in each pair within the cable from EMI from the other pairs (see Note). This potentially allows the installer to run different types of signal, for example, Ethernet + RS-485/MODBUS down the same cable without interference or 'crosstalk'. This design is found in CAT7A and some CAT6A cables. Note that mixing signal types in one cable can be problematic, so should be viewed as a contingency until proven to work.

Note: It should be noted that the screen or braid's capacitance to Earth may affect the maximum data rates achievable in some cable types.

In addition to the shielding and screening issue, CAT cables are rated according to bandwidth:

(a) Category 5e balanced cable and connecting hardware specified up to 100 MHz in accordance with BS EN 50173-1:2018 *Information technology. Generic cabling systems. General requirements* (equivalent to Category 5e as specified in American standards);

(b) Category 6A balanced cable and connecting hardware specified up to 250 MHz in accordance with BS EN 50173-1 and enabling higher data transmission rates than Category 5e;

(c) Category 6A balanced cable and connecting hardware specified up to 500 MHz in accordance with BS EN 50173-1;

(d) Category 7A balanced cable and connecting hardware specified up to 600 MHz in accordance with BS EN 50173-1; and

(e) Category 7A balanced cable and connecting hardware specified up to 1 GHz in accordance with BS EN 50173-1.

When specifying CAT cable, take steps to verify that your supplier is providing EU Construction Products Regulation (CPR) assurance. This Regulation rates all cables manufactured after 1st July 2017 according to fire performance. Additionally, BS 6701 states that:

(a) all ICT cables to be installed below floors, behind walls or to which access is limited, shall have a minimum fire performance EuroClass of C_{ca}-s1b,d2,a2, according to BS EN 13501-6:2018 *Fire classification of construction products and building elements. Classification using data from reaction to fire tests on power, control and communication cables*; and

(b) all other ICT cables shall have a minimum fire performance EuroClass of E_{ca}, according to BS EN 13501-6, or shall meet BS EN 60332-1-2:2004+A11:2016 *Tests on electric and optical fibre cables under fire conditions. Test for vertical flame propagation for a single insulated wire or cable. Procedure for 1 kW pre-mixed flame.*

Links to further guidance can be found in Appendix C.

5.6.4 When to use shielding on smart home signal cables

Ethernet (CAT) cabling in a domestic setting should not need to have shielding if the measures described earlier in this Section have been used (with distancing especially encouraged).

However, if equipment manufacturers recommend it, shielded cable should be used. The type of shielding and the nature of the bonding to the MET should be discussed with that manufacturer and the agreement reached should be documented where possible.

A shielded cable will only afford protection from EMI if it is bonded back to the MET.

The level of EMI protection is highest when both ends of the shield are bonded in a 360 ° format.

The performance of the shield is affected by its composition, including whether it is a foil or a braid.

Many manufacturers recommend the use of a shielded cable, but do not specify the precise type or the manner in which to bond the shielding. This can create a situation where sheathed cables are used, but the sheath is not bonded. This should be avoided in any event, but there are particular reasons to shun this practice in smart homes, which are illustrated below.

Figure 5.8 illustrates a risk that could arise from having unbonded sheaths on cables. ELV devices are permitted in special locations like showers – and this is one advantage of smart homes. If segregation is not achieved, environmental conditions such as abrasion could result in Band 2 voltages being transmitted to Band 1 cable sheathing or even to the conductor. If the cables are damaged, an unbonded metallic sheath, not protected by ADS, could pick up a higher (Band 2) voltage and carry it elsewhere. This is hazardous in any location, but particularly within a shower.

Section 5 – Safety aspects of smart home design

Figure 5.8   An example of undesirable outcomes of segregation

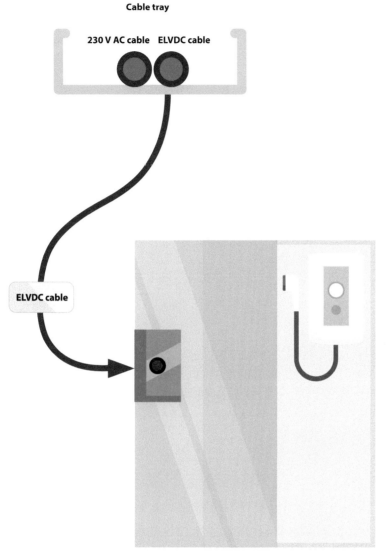

Extra attention should be given to areas including, but not limited, to the following:

(a) good workmanship, as required by BS 7671:2018+A1:2020;

(b) minimum separation distances and segregation between different energy class cables – this will be determined by the designer's own engineering judgment;

(c) all metallic sheathing should be bonded so that hazardous fault currents can be detected and disconnected by ADS circuit protection devices such as miniature circuit-breakers (MCBs) and residual-current circuit-breakers (with overcurrent protection – RCBOs); and.

(d) designers and installers should ensure that ELV power supplies for special locations such as showers satisfy both of the following criteria:

    (i) power supplies should be separated extra-low voltage (SELV) or protective extra-low voltage (PELV); and

    (ii) they should be equivalent to a safety isolating transformer.

A note on fault protection or additional protection by RCD devices:

It is a requirement of Regulation 411.3.3 of BS 7671:2018+A1:2020 that all socket-outlets rated at 32 A or less have additional protection provided by an RCD that has an operating current not exceeding 30 mA. Regulation 411.3.4 also states that within domestic (household) premises, additional protection by an RCD with a rated residual operating current not exceeding 30 mA shall be provided for AC final circuits supplying luminaires. Additional protection is also often required for cables buried or concealed in walls at a depth of less than 50 mm. In addition, BS 7671:2018+A1:2020 permits RCDs to be used for fault protection.

Final circuits used to provide power for specialist smart home equipment, for example, dimmers and power supplies, must use the appropriate type of RCD according to Regulation 531.3.3.

Type A, Type F or Type B RCDs should be selected according to equipment manufacturers' instructions, taking into account the guidance in Annex A53, Figure A53.1, of BS 7671:2018+A1:2020.

5.7 Summary

(a) Use equipment meeting the essential requirements of the EMC Regulations 2016.
(b) Keep Band 1 and Band 2 circuits separate, in accordance with BS 7671:2018+A1:2020. Separate power and data/control cabling where possible.
(c) Create functional earthing and bonding as far as is practical and cost-effective.
(d) Follow manufacturers' advice where possible. There may be uncertainty – for example, a conflict between different manufacturers' advice. Your default position is to comply with appropriate regulations, including BS 7671:2018+A1:2020.

Note that techniques to implement earthing and bonding, as this applies to smart homes, cannot be adequately covered in this Guide. Those requiring more depth should see the IET *Code of Practice for Connected Systems Integration in Buildings*, particularly Section 5. Other resources can be found in Appendix C.

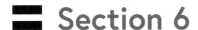 **Section 6**

Smart home infrastructure

This Section introduces and explains how smart homes are arranged, with reference to the following:

(a) cabling;
(b) wireless signals;
(c) devices;
(d) power supply; and
(e) cyber security.

6.1 How the smart home installer job is different to the electrical installer job

6.1.1 Lifespan of the installation

Electrical installers commonly encounter 40-year-old traditional copper/brass/plastic systems that function perfectly. That is unlikely to be the case with smart home installations.

The structured cabling discussed in Section 2 should remain serviceable for at least as long as traditional systems, but the smart elements – software, processors and devices – are likely to need maintenance, upgrades and replacement over the lifetime of the structured cabling.

The electrical installer should keep this in mind and design to facilitate. This is known as 'future-readying'.

Note: While Ethernet cables will remain serviceable, transmission speeds will decrease over time due to degradation of the insulation. Buying good quality cables, and careful installation, will reduce the rate of degradation.

6.1.2 Complexity of the installation

A smart home has:

(a) more components;
(b) more integration with other systems; and
(c) more networked devices, requiring new considerations for their cyber security.

6.2 Compatibility

As discussed in Section 2.7, not all systems and devices are compatible or interoperable. There is still misunderstanding about compatibility across the smart home industry, particularly amongst homeowners, but even amongst professionals. This extract from the IET *Code of Practice for Connected Systems Integration in Buildings* highlights the confusion created by assuming that two devices using Ethernet connectors and accessories will be able to talk to one another:

Ethernet networks

Note: Just because two devices may both have an Ethernet socket, enabling them to be physically connected together, they will only be able to communicate if both devices are also running software that contains the necessary application-layer protocols to enable useful communication; i.e. they must both 'speak the same language' in terms of their functions and interfaces.

Check with equipment manufacturers that the types of network hardware that you intend to install are compatible with the devices that are present in the project building. For example, a Layer 3 switch may prevent some devices, such as those that update their configuration via UDP multicast messages, from properly functioning.

It may, however, be the case that some degree of interoperability has been created by the different manufacturers or a third party.

As the designer, you will be accountable for the system's performance, including any issues with interoperability, even if they are outside of your control.

Your designed system might contain interoperable devices from different manufacturers. If one updates their software and the other does not, this could make them effectively incompatible. In the eyes of the client, that is your fault and you must fix it.

Electrical installers should seek manufacturers' advice before committing to a design that requires interoperability between products from different manufacturers. It is also worth checking about backwards compatibility of devices from the same manufacturer.

6.3 Topography (layout) of physical components

Telling an experienced electrical installer where to put a thermostat is clearly unhelpful. The question of where to put a dozen thermostats in the same house, however, does require some consideration.

Taking this situation as an example, to achieve truly smart heating, each zone should be individually controlled. This multiplies the factors to be considered:

(a) more locations means more things to avoid: over radiators, behind bookcases, out of sunlight, not where a picture is going, etc.
(b) householders may want the thermostats to be inconspicuous.
(c) more zones means more choices. Turning on central areas like landings might be seen as a good way of warming bedrooms gradually in the mornings, while warming up the UFH screed might be seen as good in the winter, but undesirably hot in the summer.

A job an electrical installer might have done a hundred times, positioning a thermostat, could thus become confusing and challenging within a smart home installation – if it is not planned for.

In practice, you will probably install sensors rather than thermostats, and these can be very small. Should you choose a manufacturer that allows this, or does the client want something chunky and recognizable?

Figure 6.1 Different types of sensor (Reproduced by permission of Loxone)

Pipe sensor

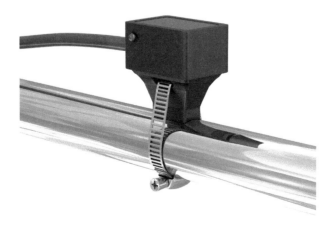

Section 6 – Smart home infrastructure

1-wire chip sensor suitable for hiding in back boxes

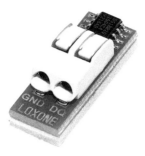

Probe sensor suitable for UFH

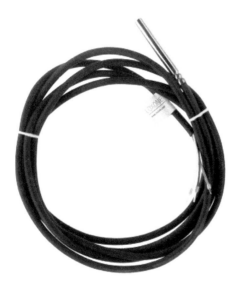

Another application that needs more thought in smart homes is motion sensing. Consider Figure 6.2, an alarm installer would naturally place a sensor to favour an access route into the room. This approach will not be satisfactory, however, if motion-triggered lighting also needs it to pick up the table where people sit, which is at the other end of the room.

A motion sensor that keeps diners illuminated, but fails to detect an intruder coming through the main window is also a failure.

Section 6 – Smart home infrastructure

Figure 6.2 Room with dining table and intrusion points at door and windows

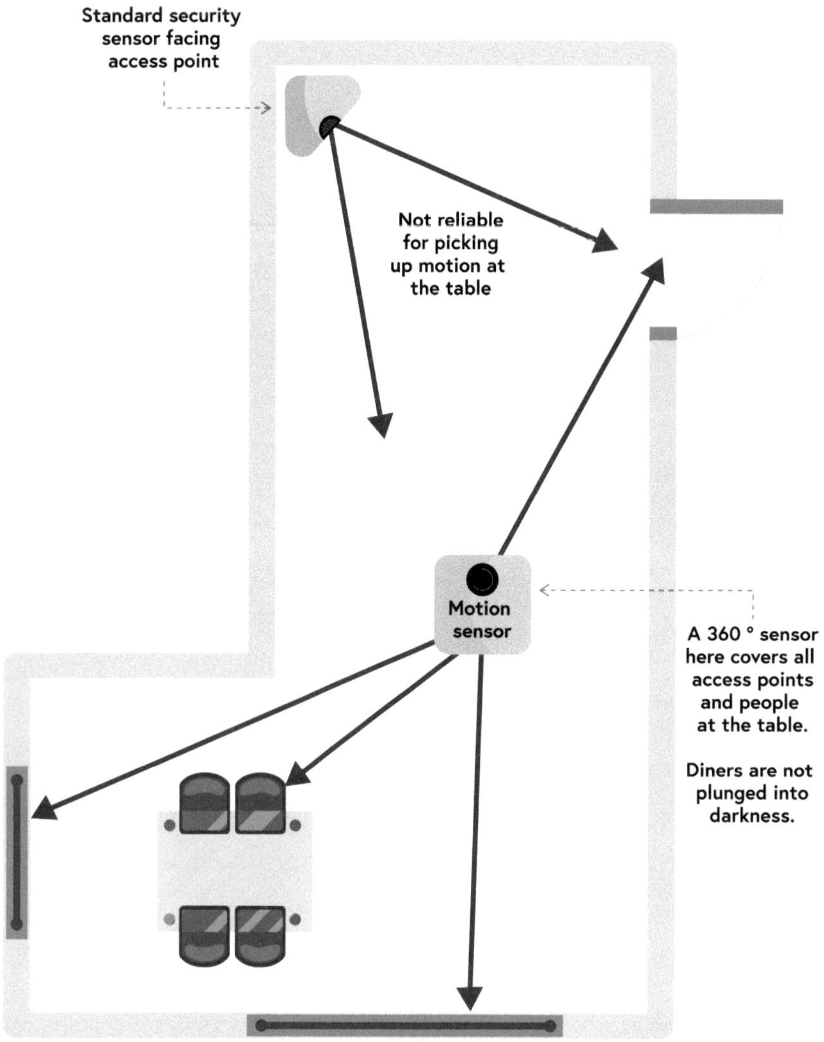

Standard security sensor facing access point

Not reliable for picking up motion at the table

Motion sensor

A 360 ° sensor here covers all access points and people at the table.

Diners are not plunged into darkness.

Key learning: Smart home components may be required to do more than one job

The 'jobs' of smart home components will be determined by the client's needs. In the example of the motion sensor, you need to know where people congregate in a room. It might be that more than one sensor is needed to cater for more than one mode of occupancy. This requirement will also depend on the flexibility of the system UI to create scenes that supplement the sensor.

Technical considerations might also flow from the different design of components. Having a temperature sensor that can be hidden in a switch back box might be convenient, but if it is isolated from the air in the room and sits against a windy cavity on a north-facing wall, it will read cold. Within a stud wall that sits on top of a UFH screed, it is likely to read warm.

It is not possible to describe all such considerations in smart home design – and layout mistakes will happen. When they do, you should review your documentation (needs analysis, consolidating needs form, functional analysis and design). What question needed to be asked or factors considered to have avoided the mistake? Add it to your process so that you can avoid making it again.

Section 6 – Smart home infrastructure

6.4   Topology (interconnections) of physical components

Once you have decided what devices are required and where they should all go, the next job is to specify how they should be connected.

The primary decision is whether the connections should be wired or wireless, as mentioned in Section 2.4. The rest of this Section provides the detail required to inform that decision.

6.4.1   Wireless connection

All wireless communication, except sound, is in a form of electromagnetic (EM) radiation. Figure 6.3 can be used as a reference to understand the EM 'landscape', including:

(a) where the radio frequencies (expanded at the top of the Figure) used for wireless signals sit within the EM spectrum (seen at the bottom of the Figure); and

(b) where the individual frequencies specified by manufacturers for their equipment (shown in labelling on the top band) sit within that band.

Figure 6.3   The EM spectrum and buildings

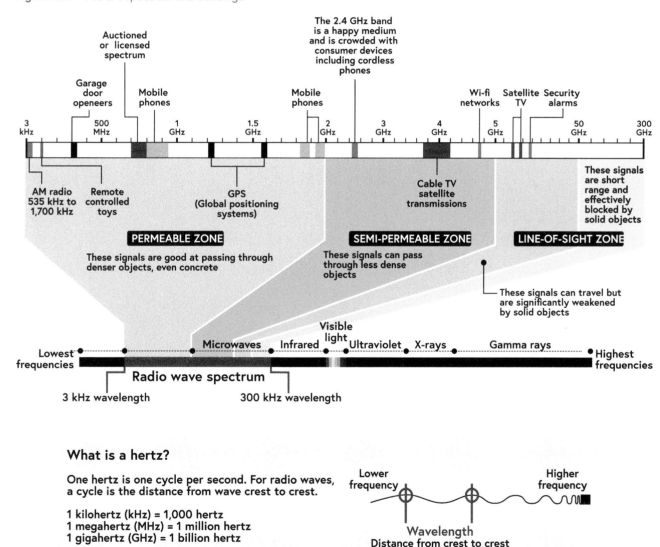

Any of the signals shown in Figure 6.3 will travel infinite distances in a vacuum and a very long distance in the Earth's atmosphere. By definition, buildings contain denser matter, so we must design for it.

Section 6 – Smart home infrastructure

Figure 6.3 also shows how frequencies can be grouped according to their ability to penetrate materials. The diagram creates three groups: a permeable zone, a semi-permeable zone and a line-of-sight zone. As we move from left to right (low to high frequency) across the frequency band, two things happen:

1. the potential for faster data speed increases; and
2. the ability to penetrate materials decreases.

Designing a smart home that relies on good signal transmission requires consideration of the signal's ability to penetrate the material of the building. Some common impediments are considered below.

Figure 6.4 shows how some materials will simply absorb the signal: high frequency signals are the most likely to be absorbed. The thicker and damper walls are, the more they block electromagnetic radiation (EMR). Lower frequencies towards the left of Figure 6.3 will tend to penetrate better than higher frequencies to the right. The absorption by the material will increase with density, thickness and dampness.

Figure 6.4   Absorption of EMR

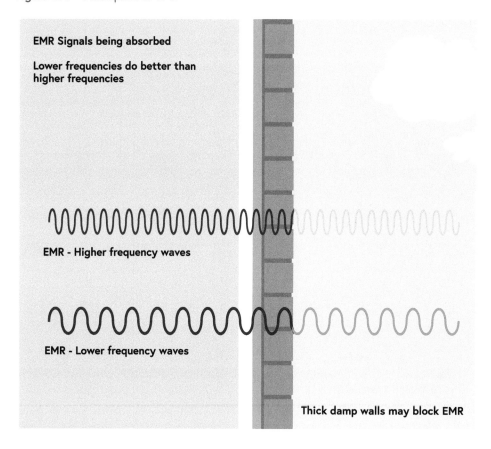

Section 6 – Smart home infrastructure

Figure 6.5 illustrates another impediment that must be considered in modern buildings, which may contain a lot of foil-backed insulation or plasterboard. Foil is reflective, and everything will bounce off it rather than go through it. The best you can hope for is that a wireless signal will ricochet to its intended destination.

Figure 6.5   Signal being reflected

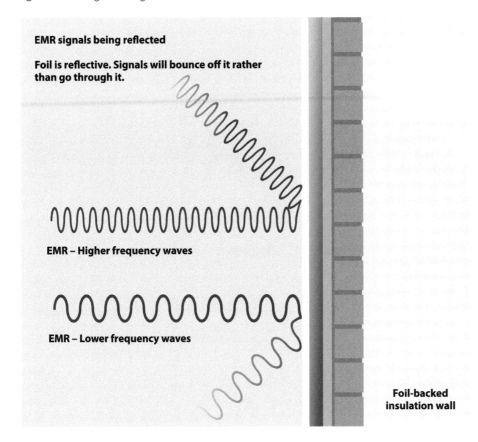

Section 6 – Smart home infrastructure

Figure 6.6 illustrates a scenario where signals get through, but are diminished. In a building that has lots of walls like this, a designer might favour devices that use lower proprietary (licensed) frequencies over internet-based (IoT) frequencies, if wireless is the only option.

Figure 6.6 EMR and permeable barriers

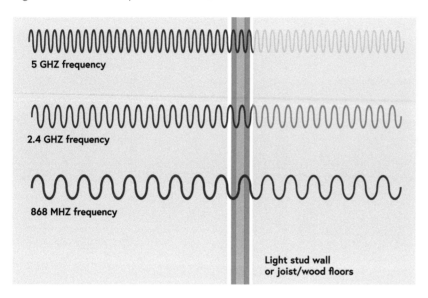

In summary, where wireless communication might be desired, a designer must assess the permeability of the environment and specify accordingly.

6.4.2 Wired signal connection

Where a device requires only AC or DC power, the manufacturer's guidelines and BS 7671:2018+A1:2020 are the principal guides.

Where the connection is for data or signals, there are other considerations. BS 7671:2018+A1:2020 and BS 6701, which were introduced in Section 5.4.2, provide guidance on such telecommunications connectivity.

Manufacturers' guidelines should also be consulted for telecommunications connectivity. It is likely that such guidelines will assume technical knowledge that you will not have encountered as a standard electrical installer. We therefore provide a summary below of the telecommunications topology you may encounter in smart homes.

6.4.3 Star wiring

Star wiring is a slightly ambiguous concept that is central to the approach taken when wiring a smart, as opposed to a traditional, home. Figure 2.25 illustrated the difference between traditional 'daisy chain' wiring from a DB and the 'star wiring' we expect to utilize in a smart home from an HE.

There is a step change in control and adaptability when you star wire.

Section 6 – Smart home infrastructure

Figure 6.7, which takes a close look at lighting, is a good way of illustrating the difference.

Figure 6.7 Traditional single-feed (top) versus star-wired central hub (bottom)

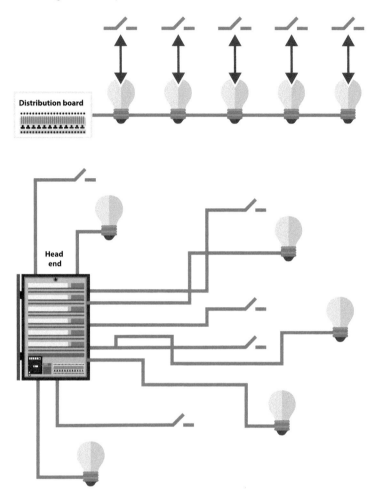

With a traditional single feed, your only option for control from the hub, in this case, the DB, is on or off for all five luminaires.

With star-wired, from the hub, the following applies:

(a) you can control all five luminaires independently;
(b) any switches connected directly to the HE might optionally be used to control any or all of those luminaires;
(c) any or all of those switches might be set up to control additional functional systems, as desired; and
(d) any or all of the luminaires might be controlled by other devices that are connected to the HE later.

Innovations in portable and 'hideable' devices, for example, IoT lamps and RF-controlled dimmers, have gone some way towards removing the need to star wire for control – and this is certainly an enabler in retrofit no-material-to-be-disturbed projects.

The star wire approach is still highly recommended for new build and wherever practical. It is more robust, affords more possibilities, minimizes device-clutter and still allows for the adoption of IoT devices, if necessary.

Section 6 – Smart home infrastructure

6.4.4 BUS topology

Clearly, star wiring means more cables back to the hub or HE. This can be more labour-intensive and expensive; however, the invention of the BUS network provides a way of communicating with multiple devices connected to a single cable.

Figure 6.8 A processor module with five switch modules

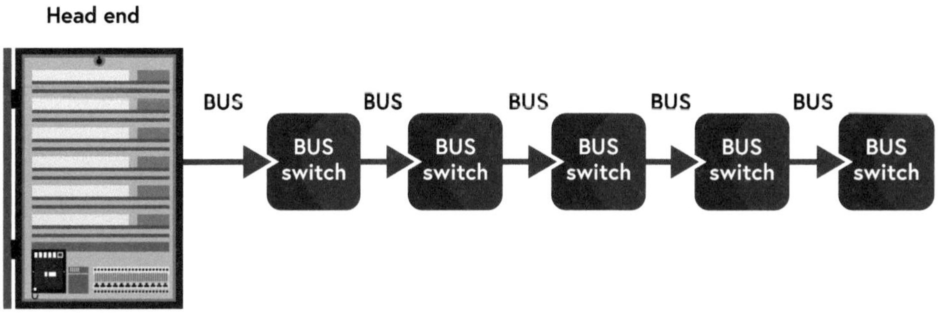

In Figure 6.8 we see that the five switches are now served by a single cable back to the HE. This provides individual control with just one cable – the best of both worlds. The devices on the BUS could just as easily be motion sensors or luminaires.

A BUS connection will necessarily rely on a communication protocol, as discussed in Section 2.9.3. This will be created or adapted by the device manufacturer and, in most cases, you will not need to understand how it works. You do, however, need to take steps to ensure that it does work, and you should consult the manufacturer to establish requirements.

Things to consider and establish when you specify a BUS connection for devices include the following:

(a) if the BUS line is cut, everything downstream and possibly upstream is effectively disconnected. Consider putting in contingency cables. A BUS is a usually a radial circuit, and not a ring, but putting in a ring return unconnected as a contingency might be worthwhile. That redundant cable should be clearly labelled as such, because connecting both ends of a BUS circuit will usually disable it.

(b) different devices have different cable lengths over which information can be relied upon, with these dependent on the cable. Establish this factor in advance of specification and ensure your design does not exceed it.

(c) BUS networks often require terminators, usually resistors, at the end of the line.

(d) increasing the number of devices on a BUS network might make it slower.

Section 6 – Smart home infrastructure

6.4.5 Ethernet

Wired local area networks (LANs) use Ethernet technology.

Ethernet LANs are star-wired. Figure 6.9 shows how devices might be connected by wire to a router.

Figure 6.9   Router with star wiring

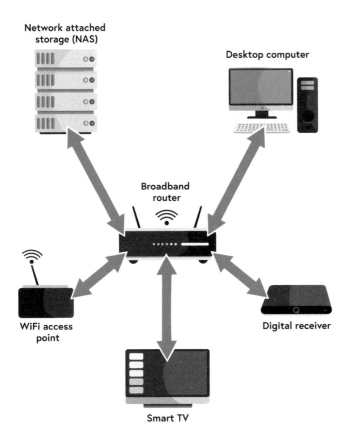

The hardware is the RJ45 socket and plug and the 4-twisted pair (Ethernet) cable.

Ethernet communications use many protocols, including TCP/IP, UDP/IP, DHCP and dozens of others, which together form the language used by the internet.

The software is potentially anything that can be written on a device that can be linked to the internet.

A lot of work has gone into developing wired and wireless protocols so that they work well alongside each other. Consumer tech manufacturers design their equipment so that it should not be necessary to know anything about a connected device other than its name on the network. A smart home engineer, however, is likely to need to know the basics of TCP/IP. Signposts to further resources on this topic can be found in Appendix C.

'Wireless' Ethernet

Section 3.2 introduced WiFi devices that can create an equivalent link (using other protocols) without data cables. This capability is now universally referred to as WiFi. As with wired Ethernet, it is a conglomeration of protocols.

Section 6 – Smart home infrastructure

Figure 6.10 shows the wired backbone of the home network (blue arrows) being extended by WiFi connection (orange arrows).

The unifying factor of the two methods, wired and WiFi, is that they both address devices by their IP number (for example, 192.168.1.20). As a rule of thumb, if a device has an IP address, it is an internet-ready device.

Figure 6.10   All devices receiving TCP/IP signals

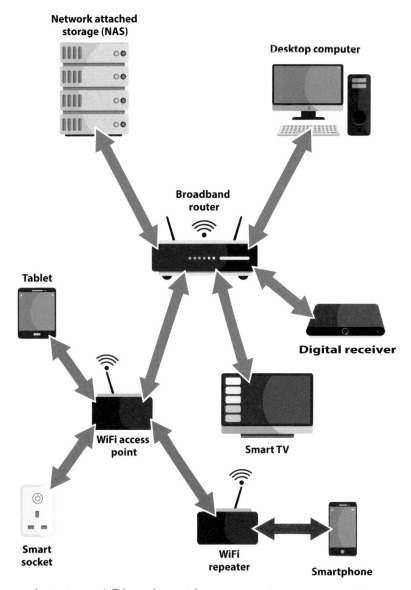

If you are designing an IoT-based smart home, your primary concern is to ensure that the Ethernet LAN is fit for purpose. Your structured cabling should include provision to support adequate WiFi cover.

Figure 6.10 has one device that is connected by a red arrow: this represents a connection that is potentially inadequate.

If we look at Figure 6.11, we see the same network, but in a physical setting. The dotted line represents the suspect connection – it may well be the case that opening and closing the doors effectively turns WiFi on and off in that room.

Section 6 – Smart home infrastructure

Scattered WiFi devices need a good Ethernet backbone – you should try to design to avoid extremities susceptible to drop-out like the smartphone in Figure 6.11. Getting an Ethernet cable to the position of the WiFi repeater so that it could be a WiFi access point would have been a better strategy. Another rescue strategy at this point could be to install a PLC plug in the poorly served room; however, remember when specifying that installed WiFi devices need to allow uninterrupted roaming to provide user satisfaction. (See Appendix C for further guidance.)

Figure 6.11   Inadequate WiFi

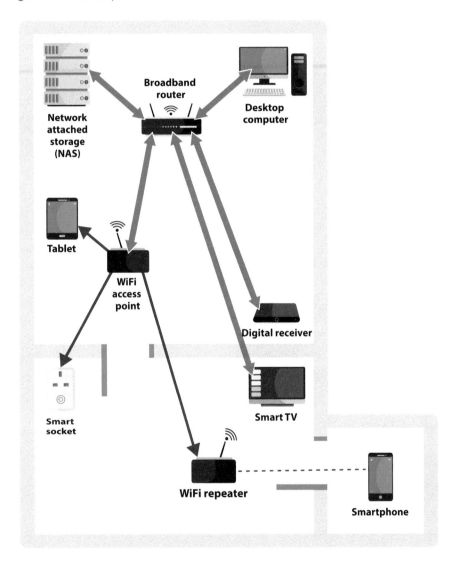

6.5   Smart home cabling

Smart homes cables may contain low voltage (LV), extra-low voltage AC (ELVAC), low voltage DC (LVDC), extra-low voltage DC (ELVDC), data, AV and Power over Ethernet (PoE). These can come in single and multi-core varieties, which can be bundled into one cable for specific applications. Fibre-optic cable can be used where products and manufacturers' guidelines permit.

Section 6 – Smart home infrastructure

Figure 6.12 shows a version of a cable format common in smart homes. It contains larger cores for ELVDC to power devices like lighting, plus twisted pairs for signals and on-board processor power.

Figure 6.12   A smart home cable (Reproduced by permission of Loxone)

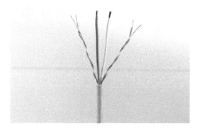

6.6   Cabling for DC power

Where standard electrical safety is concerned, BS 7671:2018+A1:2020 is the primary source of guidance. For energy efficiency, including use of DC, the basics are covered below. Signposts to other resources can be found in Appendix C.

ELVDC lighting, for example, LED strip lighting, is a common requirement in smart homes. There is also a lot of research and development into using LVDC, such as the energy output from PV inverters in the home, without turning it into AC. This means that cabling which you might assume will carry 230 V AC may quite soon be tasked to carry DC – and this has some technical implications.

In accordance with Ohm's law, lower voltages mean higher currents for the same amount of power.

For example, while LED lighting offers lower wattage per lumen, its current-drawing potential can catch you out.

Consider a 10 m colour-changing LED strip:

A load of 140 W at 14 W per metre:

- At 12 V, current I = 140/12 = 11.66 A
- At 24 V, current I = 140/24 = 5.83 A.

The current will be significantly larger than for a 230 V 140 W luminaire, which would draw 0.6 A. At a distance of 20 m from the HE, this presents a significant increase in voltage drop.

It may also need more cores – five, to be precise: red + green + blue + white + DC.

230 V AC-based assumptions and habits are liable to catch you out when working with ELVDC systems. Gather the manufacturer's data, go back to the books and work it out.

Further guidance on this subject can be found in the IET *Code of Practice for Low and Extra Low Voltage Direct Current Power Distribution in Buildings.*

Section 6 – Smart home infrastructure

6.7   Remote powering (RP) and Power over Ethernet (PoE)

Under no circumstances should Ethernet, or any other cable not approved for mains voltage, be used to carry mains (230/415 V AC) voltage.

However, it is possible for devices to receive power over telecommunications cables where all of the following conditions are satisfied:

(a) the power supply is SELV or PELV;
(b) the telecommunications cable is rated for the SELV or PELV energy it is intended to transmit; and
(c) the power supply ensures a level of fault protection equivalent to a safety-isolating transformer.

This practice is referred to as 'remote powering'. See Appendix C for signposts to further reading on this subject.

PoE is defined by the IEEE 802.3 PoE Standard, which lays out the rules for devices to receive ELVDC power through an Ethernet cable. Standard Ethernet only uses two of the four pairs, leaving one pair for +DC and one pair for –DC.

PoE is usually 24 V–48 V. The voltage can be supplied by a PoE switch at the HE or by a power-injector closer to the device to be powered. This difference is illustrated in Figure 6.13. Placing the ELVDC power injector closer to the load will mitigate the voltage drop effect described in Section 6.6, but may create extra work to house the local PoE power-injector.

Figure 6.13   Voltage supplied by a PoE switch at the HE (top) or by a power-injector (bottom)

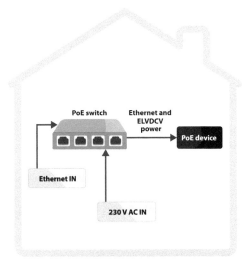

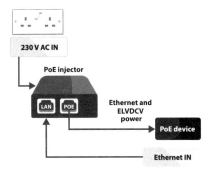

PoE supply is another area where manufacturers' guidance should be strictly adhered to. ELVDC can cause substantial heating in cables, which can result in fire. Consult BS 7671:2018+A1:2020 and the IET *Code of Practice for the Application of LED Lighting Systems* for further guidance. Always remember that bunching cables can increase the risk of dangerous heating effects, even where manufacturers' guidance has been followed.

6.8   Cabling for AV and smart home signals

Many, but not all, smart home signal cables can now be Ethernet cables.

CAT5e cable is widely considered as obsolete. CAT6A offers better bandwidth than CAT5e, as well as better capacity for PoE, due to the larger cores in the cable.

As discussed in Section 5.6.2, versions with appropriately bonded metallic screening or braiding can offer better signal integrity than unsheathed varieties.

Manufacturers' guidance should always be sought, as varying from their recommended cabling could void your warranty and support agreement.

Applications not suited to the use of Ethernet cable include, but are not limited to, amplifiers to low-impedance loudspeaker cables: these rely on low conductivity and should be matched according to manufacturers' guidance.

Fibre-optic cables may be the preferred method of connection for specialized equipment and environments.

Baluns are devices that convert balanced signals, such as those transmitted in the Ethernet twisted pair format, into unbalanced signals, such as AV over coaxial cable. Figure 6.14 shows one application where a Balun can be used to extend a high-definition multimedia interface (HDMI) signal.

Figure 6.14   HDMI extender Baluns (Reproduced by permission of Scolmore)

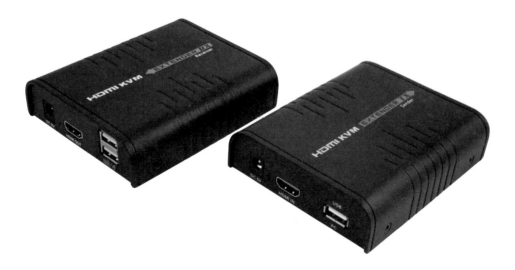

Section 6 – Smart home infrastructure

These devices can allow audio and video to be sent over Ethernet cable. Manufacturers can provide guidance on the best option to choose. To cover more eventualities, where possible, wire both Ethernet and coaxial cable to points where video and audio are required.

Signposts to guidance on structured cabling for AV can be found in Appendix C.

6.9 Cyber security

Cyber security is one of the fastest growing sectors for employment and training and is becoming a specialism in its own right.

In Section 5.3 we discussed the idea of designing for safety. It is also important in the current cyber-climate that you design for data security.

6.9.1 General Data Protection Regulation (GDPR)

The standard everyone, including electrical installers, will be held to is the GDPR. This came into force in May 2018, and much of it is aimed at companies who amass large amounts of data as part of their business. A smart home installer must hold some data to go about their business, so the GDPR does apply, but in a more limited sense.

The key themes that apply are:

(a) privacy by design (PbD):
   (i) have systems to ensure that you minimize data collection and retention;
   (ii) have systems to ensure that you gain consent from clients when you process their data.
(b) the right to erasure and to be forgotten:
   (i) this is controversial in the broadest sense of online activity.
   (ii) however, it is not controversial at all in relation to your work. If a client requests that you delete all their data, you are legally obliged to do so. Claiming you did not know you had stored it is not a defence. You therefore need systems to monitor and control where you put client information.
(c) breach notification:
   (i) companies will have to notify data authorities within 72 hours after a breach of personal data has been discovered. Data subjects (your clients) will also have to be notified, but only if the data poses a "high risk to their rights and freedoms". If you hold client information and you are 'hacked', you are obliged to inform the Information Commissioner's Office (ICO: https://ico.org.uk).

It is questionable what some of these points have to do with an electrical installer installing smart home equipment. The primary point is that as a smart home installer, you will have had access to the client's router and LAN. That alone places your activities right in the middle of the GDPR remit.

The definition of personal data according to the GDPR is "any information relating to an identified or identifiable natural person".

The following two guidelines are offered to help you:

   1. do not retain personal data beyond its original purpose; and
   2. give consumers access to and ownership of their data.

You are legally obliged to record and retain certain documents, for example, invoices for HM Revenue & Customs (HMRC) and electrical certificates for Building Control.

Section 6 – Smart home infrastructure

Arguably, your agreement with the client should specify the documents you need to file. Until they have agreed for you to keep their information, you should not do so.

With respect to the second guideline, one strategy might be to have a shared digital folder where all information relevant to the client can be kept, with joint access.

6.9.2 Bite-size cyber tips

The following tips should help when beginning a project:

(a) all the devices you use to access, process and store client data should have strong passwords.
(b) folders and/or documents in which you store client data should have strong passwords.
(c) take rigorous precautions to ensure that your passwords are controlled and audited. If you must share a password, document that it is being shared. Password changes should also be recorded by date and time.
(d) as someone trusted with client data, take extra care where and how you connect to the internet when using devices holding client data. When you look at the internet, it looks back.
(e) assess the strength of the default password. If it is weak, change it or recommend that the client considers changing it to something appropriate.
(f) when you allocate a password for a client as a user, recommend that they change the password as soon as possible.
(g) when you find a home router with default settings still on it, recommend that these are changed immediately.
(h) where you must retain network access and/or administrator access to devices on the client's network, have a written agreement to do so. Renew that agreement annually.

6.10 System requirements for data

6.10.1 Data volume

To assess storage-stress, you need to understand where information is being stored and how the storage capacity compares to the rate of storage and deletion. It may be necessary to obtain data rate statistics from manufacturers and match them to equipment and cables.

6.10.2 Design for data

With off-the-shelf stand-alone products, the traffic and storage should have been well designed for by the manufacturer. As you progress into larger, bespoke systems, the onus will fall on you as designer to ensure that all is within healthy parameters. Record and consider the storage capacity and data transfer rate of the components you specify. Check with manufacturers if you feel you may be approaching a limit.

6.10.3 Protect data

As discussed in Section 2.8, smart systems rely on intelligence. If that intelligence is compromised, the effects can be far-reaching, possibly creating a total system failure. This needs to be considered carefully: if you've installed something that controls lighting, heating and access and it has a terminal failure, where does that leave the householder on a cold day?

Ask yourself the following questions:

(a) are the parts of your system that provide intelligence protected from physical damage?
(b) are they protected from disconnection?
(c) are they supported with a contingency should either of the above occur?

Section 6 – Smart home infrastructure

(d) do you have spares? A two-week wait time on a hub processor for a fully featured smart home is likely to spoil your special relationship with the client.

(e) is the data in the server backed up? Rewriting code from memory three years after installation will not be fun and there may be learned parameters in there that you will never recover.

(f) is there a contingency connection strategy? 'Flood-wiring', i.e. putting in more CAT cables than are likely to be needed 'just in case', is becoming less favoured, but there is something to be said for identifying critical connections and putting in a spare – perhaps via another route. Figure 6.15 illustrates this contingency method.

Figure 6.15   Contingency connection for critical nodes

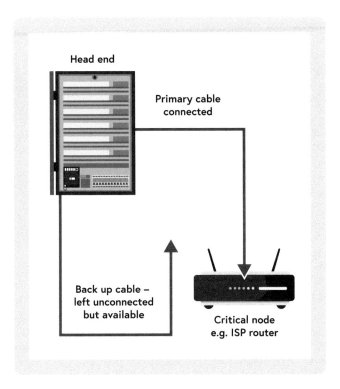

This Section has laid out some principles of smart home design to help you understand how some things are done differently to standard installation. The next step is to carry out a design that is specific to the client's needs, incorporating the equipment that best matches their requirements.

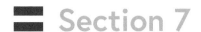 **Section 7**

Smart home design method

This Section offers guidance on how to design smart home systems – but omits discussion of how to design standard AC and DC final circuits with respect to standard characteristics such as current-carrying capacity and voltage drop. It is assumed that an electrical installer will know how to do this to comply with BS 7671:2018+A1:2020. Where the information provided in BS 7671:2018+A1:2020 is not sufficient, the designer should consult the manufacturer (and see also Appendix C in this Guide).

This Section of the Guide assumes that you have compiled the information and documentation suggested in Section 4, by use of the templates or some other means.

Documents you should have in hand before designing include:

(a) the functional analysis; and
(b) the survey and/or the plans.

If you have these, there is an option open to you that might make your job easier, which is discussed below.

7.1 Delegate design and ask a manufacturer to help

The good news for those who did a good job of the functional analysis is that any smart home manufacturer you might want to work with will be able to look at it and suggest appropriate equipment. They should also be able to deal with your subsequent questions about cabling and connections, etc.

Some manufacturers will insist that you complete their training before they will deal with you. Others will have strategies for supporting you as you take your first steps, which do not involve training. The smart home industry needs installers. There is a wide variety of training available, from manufacturers, distributors, trade associations, at industry exhibitions and, increasingly, via online courses and webinars. Large and small manufacturers alike are still working out how to support installers who are new to smart home technology.

With a good functional analysis, and a clear plan or drawing saved as a PDF, you are very well-placed to email out to 'play the field' and see which manufacturer has the best match for you and your project.

Choose wisely:

(a) check the fine print before committing to using a manufacturer's products.
(b) remember that cheapest is not always best: you will be responsible for the outcome, no matter what. With this inescapable fact in mind, it is important that you stay on track with project documentation.

7.2 Design documentation

Items that should be collated or created at the design stage include:

(a) a bill of materials (BOM);
(b) a cable schedule;
(c) a plan/drawings showing zone names and labels for cables; and
(d) a cable schematic.

7.3   A bill of materials (BOM)

This is a list of materials that will be needed for the job. It is recommended that this is compiled in a spreadsheet to make the adjustment of cost factors easier. A template for a BOM can be found in Appendix D.

Figure 7.1   Example BOM

Item	Item spec/ link	Quantity	Cost exc.	Cost inc.	VAT	Credit terms	Purchase when	Supplier	Install phase 1-5	Lead time (days)	Note
DIN Enclosure	A BB SR2 Monobloc IP65 Wal Box, Steel, Gr	1	300	360	60	Pay in advance	2 weeks before phase	Fancybox	3	14	2 man lift. Pay up front.

7.3.1   Cable schedule

A wired smart home is likely to have more cables than a standard installation. A cable schedule is essential, and should be part of your design process, rather than something you do just before you go to site. It should tell any installer or technician where each end of every cable goes.

To have any hope of success, locations should be referenced to plans or drawings. It is recommended that you use a spreadsheet for this document.

The required complexity of a cable schedule will vary with the installation. A typical cable schedule will include:

(a) a clear indication of the version (for example, 1.0, 1.1), to avoid confusion;
(b) types of cable;
(c) the labelling to be fixed to each end of the cable;
(d) the functional system of which the cable forms a part;
(e) the circuit class (for example, mains, CCTV, 24 V DC); and
(f) room for notes, for example, 'leave a lot of spare at the destination end because it might get moved'.

A cable schedule template can be found in Appendix D.

Figure 7.2   Example cable schedule

Project:										
Cable/ size	To zone/ room	Cable number	Description	Energy class	System	Emergence	Wire back to	Termination	Notes	Version
CAT 7	0/Hall	xx04	Hall motion brightness	ELVDC	Monitoring	Ceiling - Centre	HE ELVDC zone	Motion & Brightness Sensor	Void projection - keep away from joist - yellow cable	1.1
CAT 6	1 Landing	xx04	1st Landing internet	ELVDC	Wired internet	Corner opposite stair	HE: Ethernet Patch panel	Single plate RJ 45 next to power	Green cable	1.1
1.0 mm twin and earth	1/bed 1	xx08	Bed 1 downlights	230 V AC	Lighting	Ceiling - looped on to other DLs TBC	HE: switched 230 V AC zone	Downlight	Assumes LED being used - otherwise use 1.5 mm	1.1

Names and labels for cables

Start thinking about names and labelling carefully at this stage, so that all documentation (cable schedule, plans, etc.) can be consistent and intuitive. If practical, give physical items and locations names that will match their names in the UI and the householders' expectations.

7.3.2 Cable schematic

Figure 7.3 illustrates the basic idea of a cable schematic – a diagram that should give useful detail about how cables are routed.

Figure 7.3   A basic example of a cable schematic

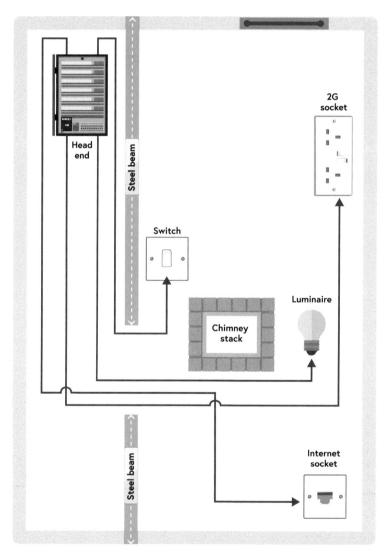

A cable schematic shows where the cables go. Achieving a detailed and helpful cable schematic for a fully featured smart home might not be practical or cost-effective, due to the number of wires. The job can thus be broken down:

(a) consider copying and annotating existing plans or drawings where available, to save time; and

(b) consider using multiple copies to illustrate separate functional groups or circuit classes, as appropriate.

Section 7 – Smart home design method

Figure 7.4 uses the same basic plan to show the routing for switches/buttons (top) and speakers (bottom).

Figure 7.4   Annotated plans to create schematics

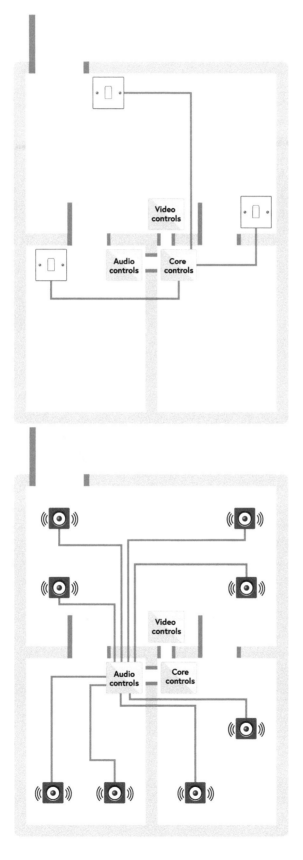

Consider using a separate 'magnifying glass' format for complex or unfamiliar systems or devices, as below.

Figure 7.5   Example schematic showing actual core runs

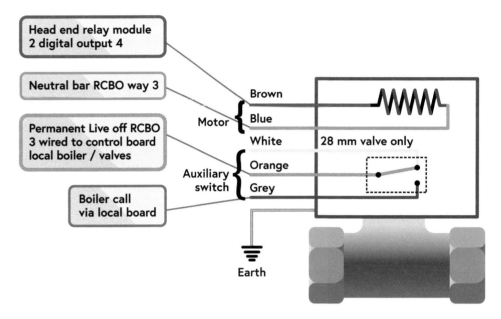

Locations on the schematic should be matched to locations in the cable schedule and to the drawings to be used on the project. Don't hesitate to 'cheat' by using diagrams provided by others.

The detail of your schematic will depend on:

(a) the environment;

(b) what the client needs;

(c) the complexity of the system; and

(d) the experience of the installation team: if this is their first experience of smart home wiring, then visual aids are a very good idea.

7.4   The difference when designing a smart home compared with a standard installation

An electrical installer designs circuits, whereas a smart home installer designs an experience.

There have been and will continue to be successful smart home designers who have very little idea of what goes on inside a cable or a device. They manage very well simply by knowing what devices can do. They employ others to deal with the technical side, while they concentrate on selling the client their 'dream home'.

An electrical installer can and should be able to do both things – but this is more challenging.

7.5 Your part in the design: where to begin

Designing all by yourself is, strictly speaking, not an option. You will need help at least in the form of technical specifications from manufacturers. Ohm's law is too blunt a tool when you need to know the maximum length a BUS circuit can be with manufacturers' sensors. Similarly, benefitting from a manufacturer's experience to understand how power consumption or voltage drop will stack up in the real world can save you a lot of work and potential problems.

Don't be afraid to ask manufacturers if your idea will work. Irrespective of the input of manufacturers in the specification of a device, you still have a major role in design – that of meeting the client's expectations.

Start from the functional analysis: an itemization by room or zone of what the householder expects. Note that a functional analysis does not include behind-the-scenes items, but just things that the client experiences. It is a good idea to transfer the functional analysis onto a plan – for one thing, this helps you to verify expectations, including locations, with the householder. Many architects include furniture in their drawings, reflecting what was discussed and agreed with the client. It is a good idea to follow their lead in this respect.

When producing drawings, the most important thing is that the client understands them. Using recognized symbols for objects will make the resources you create more useful to other trades and professions. A document containing standard audio, video and control architectural drawing symbols is listed in Appendix C. Computer-aided design (CAD) applications exist to help, but these have a learning curve which it might be best to defer until you are more familiar with smart home basics.

Figure 7.6   A functional analysis

Functional analysis for the snug:

- 4 downlights, dimmable, controlled by physical switch in room also by the system through the user interface.
- Temperature sensor linked to system – location to be confirmed
- Motion sensor linked to system – location to be confirmed. This should be able to trigger lighting if that is desired TBC.
- X1 switch by the door to control lighting and blinds
- X2 ethernet outlets behind the TV and music centre location*
- X2 RG6 Co-axial outlets behind the TV location*
- X2 speaker cables to ceiling*
- 13 A socket-outlets – number and location TBC

Figure 7.7   Plan corresponding to the functional analysis

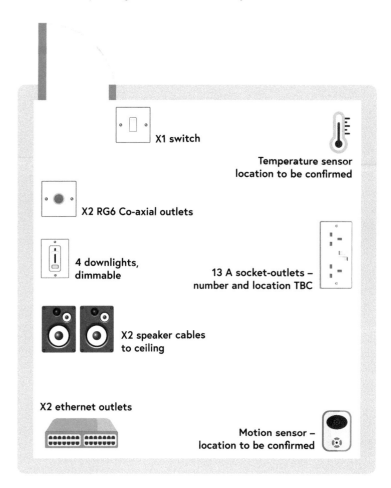

With the resources above in hand, you should now turn from facing the client to facing the building and the other trades involved in the project. You need to ask and answer every question required to ensure that the installation is safe and meets expectations. No guide could hope to walk you through all the possible questions – the next Section is simply intended to illustrate where the questions are.

7.6   A grossly simplified design method

7.6.1   Final circuits

If there are no BUS circuits, your job is to specify the appropriate cable from every device set – monitored or controlled – back to the HE. Note that a WiFi access point is a device.

Figure 7.8   Device sets (bottom) compared with a single device (top)

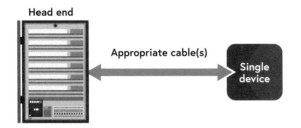

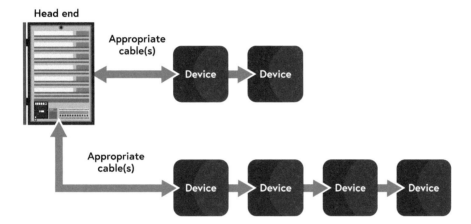

To clarify a common confusion, star-wiring necessitates a cable or cables (as per equipment requirement) to each device set – and not to each device.

In the examples shown in Figure 7.8, all three cables serve a non-BUS device set.

Assuming they are all identical devices, the cable would be the same format and the control at the HE would be the same format. The only thing that might change would be the current-handling capacity: i.e., there might be a thicker cable or higher-current control equipment for the larger set.

Where there are BUS circuits, your job is a little easier. In this circumstance, you only need one appropriate cable per BUS back to the HE, as shown in Figure 7.9. Note that Figure 7.9 also features an unconnected contingency cable.

Figure 7.9   BUS device wiring

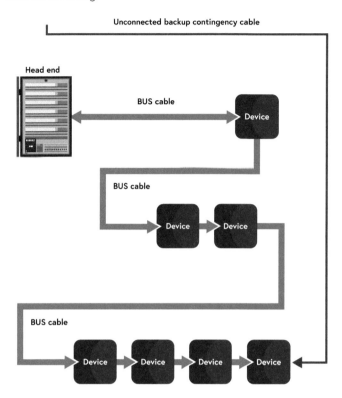

7.6.2   HE configuration

Your job is to include devices at the HE that deliver what the functional analysis promises.

Figure 7.10   A simplified HE

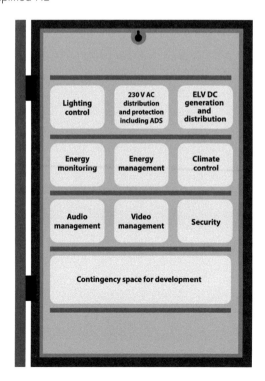

Clearly, the contents of the HE will be dependent on the design. The manufacturer should be able to tell you what is required if you gave them a good functional analysis.

7.7 Realistic questions to ask when realistically designing

In every field, the best practitioners are always learning. To help you 'keep the wheels on' while you are adapting, consider the list of example questions provided below, which a smart home designer might ask other parties involved in the project.

7.7.1 Questions to ask of manufacturers

From stand-alone consumer tech to advanced integration, manufacturers are your partners in this. They should be available to answer all your standard questions, as well as your smart questions, which might include the following:

(a) do they have guidance on how to design using their equipment? As an example, if they have a good, cost-effective device that combines a switch with a temperature sensor, that will affect how you design a system using their equipment.

(b) do they have guidance on how to wire their devices (with diagrams preferred)? For example, are you aware that all DC power supplies in an integrated system must have their negative terminals connected – and that the system is unlikely to work properly if you don't? Wiring diagrams will help you avoid potentially disastrous quirks such as that.

(c) what is the wattage/current draw of devices? This allows you to size cables and power supplies.

(d) what are the power supply options of devices? Does the power supply unit (PSU) have to be local or in the HE?

(e) how many devices can be supported per module or channel? Knowing how many devices a module or BUS can support is essential if the client requests an addition.

(f) what is the wattage/current rating/cable length of channels? Where it is not possible to state devices per channel, you should know the appropriate physical limit for that channel so that you can calculate the maximum.

(g) what is the cable required for devices? If this is specialist, the manufacturer should inform you.

(h) is there any guidance on the space, enclosure and equipment required at the HE? Running out of space can be a disaster. The manufacturers have been in this situation before, and you haven't, so take their advice.

(i) are there any specialist tools and processes that might be required for installation?

Manufacturers may have resources to help you see how components stack up against requirements. A template 'design audit' spreadsheet can be found in Appendix D. As a universal template would be very large and confusing, this simpler spreadsheet can be used and adapted instead, to start you off thinking about how to match components up in your design.

Figure 7.11   Example of a design audit

Device	Input or output	Model	Energy	Power (W)	Likely cable	Bandwidth requirement	Number of cores required	SHHE con-nection type	Number	Note
Motion sensor	Input	Danlers CEFL PIR 24VDC	ELVDC	0.1	CAT 5 or above	Low	4	Digital input	9	
Retractive switch	Input	TBC	ELVDC	0.1	CAT 5 or above	Negligible	2	Digital input	7	Get samples to show client
Temperature sensor	Input	Loxone 0-10 V indoor temperature sensor	ELVDC	0.1	CAT 5 or above	Low	3	0-10 V analogue input	8	
230 V lumi-naire set	Output	Generic	230 VAC	100	1.5 mm twin and earth	NA	3	5 A relay	6	
LED RGBW strip <10	Output	24 V generic	24 VDC	150	1.5 mm core flex	NA	5	DMX controller	1	
IP Camera	Input	HIK vision IPC-T240H	12 VDC	5W	CAT 5 or above	2 Mbps	Ethernet	RJ45	3	

Crucially, be prepared to go back to confirm that the design matches the client's expectations. They should have a copy of the same functional analysis you are working off, to leave no room for doubt.

Finally, consider asking for help from the manufacturer when figuring out stuff that you 'know', but are not 100 % sure about in the new context. This situation is likely to arise. Remember that you might be putting business their way, so insist on good customer service, and if this is not on offer, consider alternative suppliers.

7.7.2 Questions to ask of the client

As you develop your design, keep asking yourself if it matches the client's expectations.

If you are in doubt, check first with the manufacturer, then with the client.

Common zones of client uncertainty include:

(a) the positioning of devices; and
(b) cost.

Positioning of devices

Electrical installers will know how interesting it can be to plan multi-switch lighting in areas like stairs or landings, or to use motion sensing and switch combinations. People understandably don't know how they are going to use switching until they live in a space. A smart home is a giant multi-switch combination device, so clients are very unlikely to understand in advance how it will all work with them living in it.

As an example, if a householder opts for motion sensors controlling lighting, then positioning the switch plates as they would be in a traditional house is going to result in a lot of redundant switch plates (Figure 7.12 explores this situation). With traditional design, an electrical installer would probably specify a switch at each entrance point, with some capacity for two- and three-way switching.

With the introduction of automated lighting based on presence detection, the requirement for switches is reduced.

In the instance shown in Figure 7.12, one switch point by the bi-fold door would probably be sufficient, being near the gathering features and available to control outdoor lights too.

Figure 7.12   Multi-entrance room with gathering features

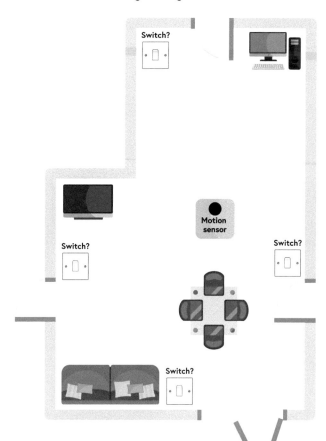

Cost

Clients for whom cost is no object are exceedingly rare. On the other hand, smart home systems that exceed the client's and designer's initial ballpark estimate are exceedingly common.

This should not and need not be a zone of uncertainty. Keep your BOM up to date and keep an eye on the bottom line in relation to the client's budget. If it starts to look too costly, talk to your client about whether they want to compromise on the design. Is there another manufacturer who could offer the same functional specification at lower cost – and what are the implications of that lower cost? Give the client the information they need to make an informed decision. They may choose to find the money once you have explained the benefits.

7.7.3   Questions to ask of the architect

Where should the HE go?

You might need to ask if space can be found for the HE, and where they think it should go. They might know, for example, that the attic will be cool and will be able to create time-saving and future-ready duct space while the design is still fluid.

For a reasonably well-featured smart home, think along the lines of the HE enclosure shown in Figure 7.13. Clearly, an enclosure of this size is not going to go in a kitchen wall cupboard or in the hall above a mirror, and you should ensure that this is understood early on in the process.

Figure 7.13 A 3 x 690 mm rail enclosure (Reproduced by permission of Loxone)

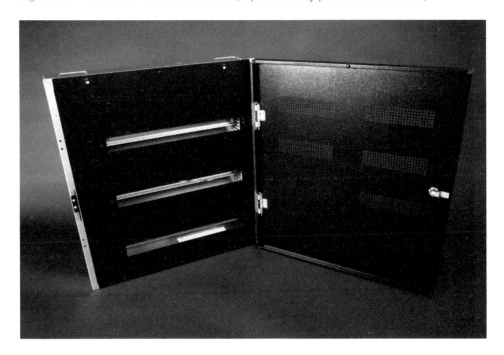

What about lighting?

Is the architect aware of the increased range of lighting that you can offer? Figure 7.14 illustrates the potential for using colour and concealed lighting that traditional installation might struggle to provide.

Figure 7.14 An example of smart home lighting design

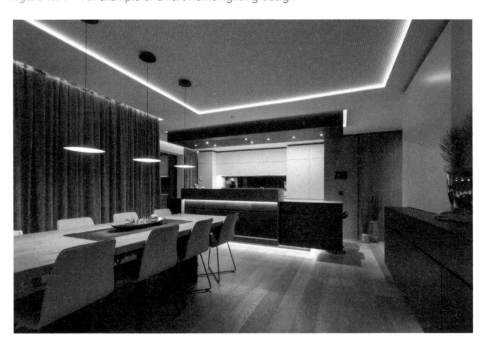

Smart home technology?

Does the architect feel that there are any elements of the building that would benefit from smart home technology? For example, they might feel that light-level sensitive shading would enhance the top floor, which is to be made of glass (and which you might well not have noticed is to be made of glass on the plan). Don't be too proud to pick up ideas from others, particularly if they are experienced designers.

Cables?

Is the architect aware of the increased volume of cables that will be involved, particularly at the HE? Do any structural alterations need to be made?

7.7.4 Questions to ask of other trades

Builder

(a) Can space be found for the HE?
(b) Are they aware of the delicacy of signal cables like CAT cable, and their bending radius?
(c) Are they happy to accommodate lighting ideas, perhaps with power supplies that might need to be local to light sources?
(d) Are they aware of the increased volume of cables that will be involved, particularly at the HE? Do any structural alterations need to be made?

Plasterer

(a) Are they happy to plaster the detail required around lighting like that shown in Figure 7.14?

Joiner

(a) Are they aware how much space you might need for access and junctions when installing bespoke luminaires?

It might be that the joiner will need to design to follow you. Access for maintenance might also be required, so alternatives to nails should be considered.

Heating engineer

(a) Are they aware of any non-standard heating controls you are supplying? Motorized valve actuators are still not commonplace on radiators and they are not likely to require a traditional UFH manifold controller in a smart home.
(b) Do you need to discuss a commissioning procedure? If you are installing an app-based UI, are they happy to use it or should you provide a manual means of control for their benefit while they are commissioning?

Kitchen fitter

Do they understand that if Ethernet outlets are specified behind units, these must remain accessible?

7.7.5 Questions to ask of trade and professional organizations

Certification bodies such as Elecsa, NICEIC and NAPIT Certification have technical helplines for their registrants. Professional bodies such as the ECA, CEDIA and the IET also have technical helplines for members. Don't be shy if you need a second opinion. These organizations are eager to keep up to date with what is happening in the smart home industry and your questions will help them to keep abreast of developments and adapt their services accordingly.

7.8 The electrical installer as the (energy-efficient) smart home installer

Much of the tone of this Guide is cautious, advising you, the new entrant, on how to take steps to hedge against mistakes.

Caution when dealing with new materials and systems is no bad thing – but it should be remembered that an electrical installer brings existing skills and knowledge to smart home installation that a designer with no electro-technical training lacks. Those skills and knowledge could provide an advantage when planning systems that consume and manage significant electrical power.

In particular, as an electrical installer, you have the core knowledge and skills that are essential to apply smart home technology to the most important and most recently mandated aspect of electrical design – namely, energy efficiency.

BS 7671:2018+A1:2020 continues to expand in scope in line with European and international standards. These provide a framework for the energy efficiency of electrical installations, allowing clients to stipulate the level of energy efficiency and production, for example, microgeneration, that they want their installation to achieve. Much of the content is aimed at commercial and industrial installations, but some categories might trickle across to domestic installation, and are discussed below.

The efficient placement of DBs

An electrical installer is best placed to assess loads and suggest the best position for DBs, to minimize cable losses.

Electrical distribution wiring system efficiency

An electrical installer is best placed to design the cable layout to minimize voltage drop and hence increase efficiency. Sub-distribution boards may be the best way, in which case the controls that might once have all been at the HE for convenience should be distributed to increase energy efficiency.

Types of controls to avoid wastage

A smart home is packed with controls that can minimize wastage. An electrical installer who properly understands the smart controls that conserve energy and improve efficiencies will perform best when positioning and configuring them.

Provision of energy measurement

Energy supplier smart meters offer the means to measure the net usage and generation of everything downstream. Energy supplier smart meters and in-home technology business models will continue to develop alongside one another. Whilst it is likely that more devices will become smart-meter-compatible, structured cabling that safeguards the ability to meter in either scenario is the best option. An electrical installer is best placed to ensure this occurs.

Types of loads that can be switched off without impacting safety and usability

'Types of loads' can be learned from a list. However, being able to design a system that allows those loads to be isolated requires the knowledge and expertise of an electrical installer. Grouping circuits to prioritize for energy efficiency is known as 'energy meshing', with star wiring a major facilitator of this. For example, SETS, as discussed in Section 1.6.5, might usefully be wired as a mesh to match microgeneration, or light sources might be placed near natural light on one circuit and attuned to light-harvesting.

Electrical system energy management

Consider:

(a) microgeneration;
(b) battery energy storage;
(c) EVs, including vehicle-to-home and vehicle-to-grid energy transfer; and
(d) SETS.

All of these involve current transfer greater than that which can pass through a UK 3-pin plug, which means that your skills as an electrical installer are needed. The smart home of tomorrow must have energy efficiency designed into it – and an electrical installer is required to make that happen. Central to that requirement is the fact that the electrical installer must understand and be able to work with smart home technology.

See Appendix C for signposts to further resources on energy efficiency in buildings.

7.9 Summary

As an electrical installer, you know how to carry out electrical installation. To be in control of a smart home installation:

(a) follow guidelines to produce a good functional analysis;
(b) use the functional analysis to identify good manufacturers with which to partner; and
(c) stay on track with the process and documentation described in this Guide.

The central component of your design will be your cable schedule, referenced to locations on plans. Other items may include:

(a) a schematic;
(b) a BOM;
(c) product literature; and
(d) a timeline.

The key design criteria for the HE at this stage is knowing how much wall you need for the enclosures. Remember to seek manufacturers' guidance wherever necessary.

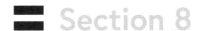

Section 8

How to propose and install smart home equipment

This Section considers how and why the proposal and installation for a smart home project might be different to a proposal for a standard installation, covering:

(a) documentation;
(b) procedures; and
(c) equipment.

8.1 What is at stake?

A smart home installer designs an 'experience' for the client, and not just a collection of circuits. That experience will be ongoing, through the installation and into support and maintenance.

Your offer to the client will be a proposal, setting out a way to deliver what they have asked for using the technology you have specified. Where installations are more complex and less familiar, the potential for misunderstandings increases. Even a superb design and installation can lead to a bad experience for those involved if the proposal, as the client receives it, is flawed. Section 8.2 expands on the extra considerations for smart home proposals.

8.2 Extra considerations for smart home proposals

1. **More elements**

2. **More technologies**

3. **More systems to be integrated**

    Items 1–3 sit together as a set of things that make the job more complicated. The 'KISS' approach ('keep-it-simple-stupid') is an option you forfeit when you make the transition to smart home installation. These are not considerations you are likely to stipulate in your proposal: the client needs to feel you have the measure of these things. However, every part of your proposal needs to take account of these facts.

4. **More liaison with other trades over detail and timings**

    The technology can lead you into processes you have not experienced before. You may need to get answers and communicate with other trades at different stages in the project. Consider stipulating this in your agreement.

5. **More tie-in to clients**

    Hope for the best, but prepare for the worst in your proposal.

    Your design could be superb, but if your client's expectations are not met, in any sense, and for whatever reason, you could be in trouble even if it's not your fault.

    With an open-ended agreement for support, the client might legally call on your time for free, forever (or at least for a very long time).

    This situation tends to resolve itself more readily in standard electrical installation. The technology is mature and anyone can find another electrician – and so a client and installer can in most cases drift apart if they want to. If you are the only installer within a 70-mile radius who is trained for a specific brand, this is not so easy.

    Therefore a definition and limitation of 'support' is required in your proposal. This should be put in a positive way; the aim is to create a structured and mutually beneficial relationship.

6. **More tie-in to manufacturers, due to specialized equipment**

7. **Higher liability for warranty**

Items 6 and 7 go back to the choices you made in your design. Consider that the best system for the project might not be compatible with any other system. There might be a long wait for a failed part that might need to be paid for in advance.

You are likely to be specifying and re-selling components that are both more expensive and more crucial than you are accustomed to in traditional installation. Are the terms of warranty made clear to the client? Developers have a five-year obligation to service the homes they sell and it is suggested that smart home proposals should reflect that timeframe. Such considerations need to be factored into your proposal, including costings.

8. **More accountability for outcomes**

As a smart home installer, you will be installing equipment and programming for the monitoring and subsequent control of all operated systems in a house. This can make you more accountable for what happens in that house than you would be for putting in a traditional system. Many electrical installers will have had tense conversations about a defrosted freezer due to a tripped RCD – there is potentially much more scope for such conversations with a smart home. Ideally, your design should rule out all such possibilities, but your proposal should consider that unexpected things do happen. Consider your insurance: is there a need to review existing cover?

8.3   Reasons to continue

A logical question to ask at this point is 'why bother?' to do something that increases exposure as described here. Some people might choose not to, and this could be the right decision for them.

The benefits of smart home installation were discussed in Section 1, but as a reminder for those still wondering whether to dip their toe in – or dive in – the motivation to do so is likely to be increased opportunities, including:

(a) higher profits on specialized projects;
(b) ongoing revenue from maintenance and support; and
(c) creating better buildings in terms of lifestyle, looks and sustainability.

8.4   The contract or agreement

A contract can be verbal. However, a verbal contract for a fully featured smart home is not 'smart' and it is strongly recommended that you have a written contract.

Remember that any access to the home network requires permission, to comply with the GDPR. Therefore, the document-free smart home job no longer exists. However, that does not mean that you have to throw lengthy documents at every job. Instead, you should differentiate the proposal to the job. This Section gives guidance on what needs to be included in your proposal.

8.4.1   Proposal elements could include

1. **Functional analysis**

Every proposal should have this upfront.

It should only be as complex as the project requires.

The client's agreement that it reflects their needs should be implicit in their signing the contract.

With the functional analysis signed off, it serves as a checklist at the end of the job.

2. **Relevant information on warranty terms for all equipment to be supplied**

Including all the warranty literature at this point is not appropriate. Framing the key points is, however, essential. For standard items, retrospective reference to 'manufacturers' terms and conditions' might be reasonable. Where a single item might be worth more than £1,000, and be crucial to the operation of a system worth £20,000, it is fair and advisable to set out the terms before the client signs.

3. **Outline of logistics**

For a job such as installing a smart thermostat, this is likely to involve nothing more than naming a day and asking that the airing cupboard be cleared.

For a fully featured smart home, there will be more to think about and this ought to be set out in an accessible way to the client. Gantt (generalized activity normalized time table) charts and a communication plan would be excessive at this point, but it might be constructive to note in writing that you need the co-operation of others to do a good job.

4. **Outline of finance requirements**

Different contractors have different preferences as to how to frame their price to the client. Clients have their own preferences too. Your experience and your instincts will guide you on how to structure the price.

As a baseline, while you are new to this, it is recommended that you:

(a) reference the price to the functional analysis.

(b) include an outline of key components, some of which may be generic. Consider adapting your BOM to allow for an easy cut-and-paste here, to save time.

(c) phase payments. Set out clearly when you need payments, quantified and referenced to identifiable milestones in the project. Keep it positive, but make clear the consequences of non-payment in your agreement.

5. **A statement regarding limitations to liability**

As discussed in Section 5.3, there are some extra considerations in this area. No-one in the smart home industry has all the answers to this situation yet, as it is still evolving.

Stop and think about what could happen. For example: who is responsible for the router/home network after you have finished your job? If the client's internet service provider (ISP) sends them a new router and they lose remote access, are you responsible for the consequences? If an auto-update of a smartphone disrupts connectivity, are you responsible? Many things that are outside of your control can cause malfunction and expense and you should consider to what degree your proposal should place limits on this liability.

6. **Provision for amendments to requirements**

Make it clear that your client can still talk to you if they wish to alter their requirements.

Explain how that will work and how it might affect costs.

7. **Costed maintenance schedule options**

Not mentioning this in a proposal for a system that will require technical maintenance might justifiably attract the criticism of 'hidden costs'. It could even be the cause of dispute. Outline the main elements (for example, software updates) and the benefits and costs of maintenance where this is likely to be required.

8. **GDPR requirements**

Make sure your proposal communicates the requirements of the GDPR in the context of your work.

8.4.2 Selling

Once you have established the particulars of your offer, don't forget to sell it! Find ways to emphasize the benefits of the system you are offering. Ask manufacturers if they have promotional resources which you might reference or include with your proposal.

8.5 How to install a smart home system

Once a proposal is accepted and the work has been ordered, the installer needs to organize the installation. This Section provides pointers to elements that might require special attention if you are unaccustomed to smart home installation, and resources to help you organize.

8.5.1 How smart home installation is different to standard installation

Before we discuss how to plan for installation, we should recap some aspects that make smart homes more of a challenge:

(a) many cables go to different places. Switch cables and cables for luminaires will typically all go back to the HE.
(b) many cables are different. Ethernet and novel cables, as dealt with in Sections 5.6.2 and 6.6–6.9, for example, require special considerations.
(c) there is more information to process about all the new equipment and the protocols required to make it work.
(d) traditional controls like rocker switches and dials disappear – to be replaced by gadgets such as detectors, buttons and screens.
(e) there is more thinking required about how to time things and fit all the new processes in.
(f) cable segregation becomes more of a challenge, as discussed in Section 5.5.
(g) impeccable cable-labelling becomes a matter of survival! There will be more cables, which will make the hunting down of mystery cables harder.

An experienced electrical installer has 95 % of the skills required to do the physical installation of smart home devices. The trick is to prepare yourself for that extra 5 %.

If you have done a good job of the documentation so far, then most of your preparation for this is done.

8.6 Documentation

Documents that should be collated or created before you install include:

(a) the functional analysis; and
(b) the proposal.

Remember that your role is to design an experience that meet expectations. These two documents are the measure of your success in the client's eyes, whether you meet the requirements of the regulations or not.

You should know your documents extremely well and keep them handy to check. If this sounds too onerous on top of the normal installation process, then think seriously about hiring more people. If you can't hire more people, then be careful as to how much you take on.

8.6.1 A timeline

A timeline is anything that identifies the sequence of events. Figure 8.1 illustrates some ways of creating a timeline. This could be a simple list, a graphical line with events on it, or a Gantt chart.

Figure 8.1   Example of timeline methods

Number	Activity	Week
1	Get 1st fix materials	0
2	1st fix	1
3	1.5 fix - pre-boarding	4
4	2nd fix	6
5	Commission	8
6	Handover	9

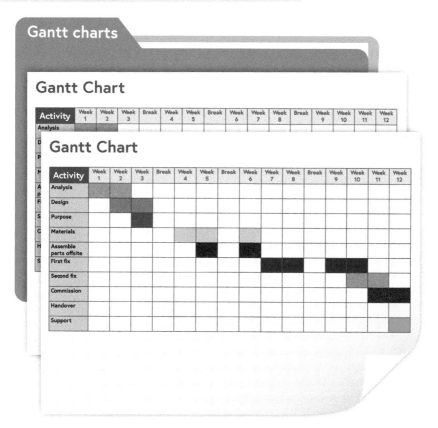

Signposts to further reading on timelines can be found in Appendix C.

Any of these methods can be as simple or complicated as required. You should have some form of timeline for every smart job you do. This habit will help you stay on track in complicated installations and will help you identify and plan for opportunities further down the road, for example, support contracts.

A timeline can remind you when you need to get extra resources to site, like specialist labour and materials, whilst you are busy dealing with all the new wires.

8.6.2 The bill of materials (BOM)

The BOM, described in Section 7.3, should be linked with the timeline, because your purchasing is more likely to be phased. Having a system where you have already identified when payments need to be made to enable you to make purchases can be a lifesaver if you are distracted by a demanding and unfamiliar installation.

8.6.3 The cable schedule

Described in Section 7.3.1, you will have collated the things required for the cable schedule at the design stage. Make them available to anyone with any responsibility for cabling.

(a) Record any changes to the cable schedule on your master copy.
(b) Make sure that everyone uses it to label things appropriately as they progress.
(c) Use the schedule to track completion.

8.6.4 The cable schematic

This is drafted at the design stage (and described in Section 7.3.2). Be prepared to adapt or explain the schematic to your team or other trades as the situation on the ground unfolds (and things materialize in unexpected places). Keeping your installation sound and safe is the priority. If you must move things to accommodate, keep a note on your master copy.

8.6.5 Manufacturer technical/installation/reference materials

These materials are quite likely to form the thickest section of your project folder. They should be accessible on-site with you from day one.

These materials contain the detail of the equipment, which is complex and unfamiliar. Do not make assumptions – instead, check all details. On-site circumstances can change cabling requirements, so have the literature to hand to verify that adjustments are compliant.

Work up your own design sketches as appropriate, to complement these materials. Doing this can confirm specifics in your own head and illustrate to others how things will fit together. They can also inform and be part of your risk assessments or method statements.

8.6.6 Risk assessments and method statements

Risks assessments and method statements are required for all jobs, and required in writing with the documentation if there are five or more employees, to comply with CDM guidelines.

As discussed in Section 5.3, having a system that supports you in developing your scope and that satisfies health and safety requirements should be seen as a good thing.

A suggested template for method statements can be found in Appendix D.

Figure 8.2   An example task-specific method statement

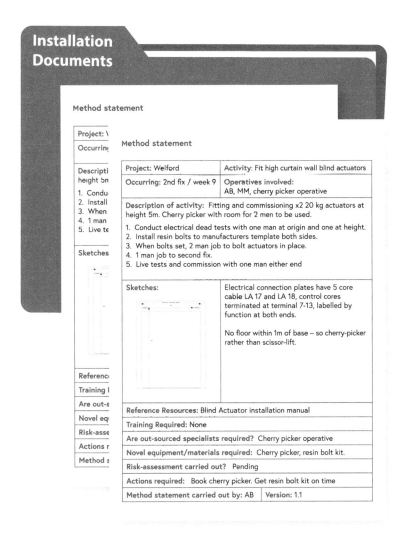

You should get into the habit of creating method statements and making them the core of your health and safety documentation. They have all sorts of benefits, including allowing you to identify when you need extra help.

8.7   Installation

8.7.1   First fix

Labelling

Every cable should have, as a minimum, both ends permanently and clearly labelled to correspond to the cable schedule.

Pulling cables

Pulling cables is not something an electrical installer needs coaching on, but you should bear in mind that signal cables tend to be more delicate than mains cables, because their insulation, sheathing and cores are typically thinner.

Bear in mind these three pointers:

1. try to minimize strain as you are pulling signal cable;
2. pay close attention to minimum bend radii, as this can cause signal degradation; and
3. avoid compressing cables with cable ties or clips, as this can cause signal degradation.

Installers should comply with BS 7671:2018+A1:2020 with respect to the fixing, routing and support of all cables. Regulations 521.10 and 527.2 of BS 7671:2018+A1:2020 describe the principles for installation and sealing of holes. Bear in mind that although it is likely that fewer cables will carry 230 V AC, it is likely that there will be more cables and more penetrations of the building fabric.

The smart home HE

Don't trim your cables too short. As a rule of thumb, leave 3 m, as shown in Figure 8.3, from the point of entry to the planned enclosure. When you have done several the same, you will be able to conserve cable – until then, leave your options open.

Figure 8.3   Example of likely enclosure

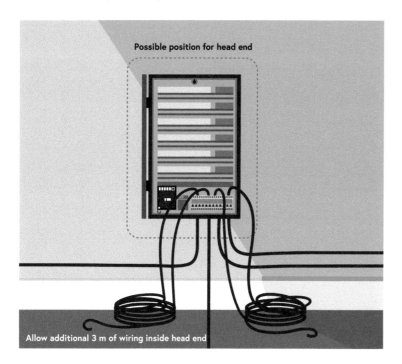

8.7.2   Second fix

Consider off-site assembly

(a) Smart home components can be expensive and sensitive; and
(b) Terminations can be intricate and time-consuming.

Consider assembling some parts off-site, away from noise and dust, to save trouble.

Follow manufacturers' guidelines

Where you are working with unfamiliar smart home equipment, your primary resources are the manufacturers' guidelines. These should have been gathered and considered at the design stage.

An electrical installer does not need to be told how to read a manual. However, you should remember that the best resource in any technical information is often the telephone number to call when the guidance is found to be lacking. Don't be too shy or stubborn to call it: the consequences of not calling could be very expensive when dealing with smart home technology.

Identify and source training requirements in advance

Smart home manufacturers are quite rightly not going to be interested in telling you how to terminate CAT cables in an RJ45 plug. Most electrical installers will know how to wire a CAT5e plug as shown on the left in Figure 8.4: but how well would they cope with the CAT7a plug on the right, without appropriate instruction and practice?

Figure 8.4   A standard CAT5e plug (left) and a CAT7a plug (right)

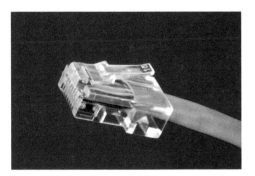
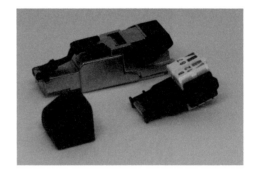

Similarly, wiring a patch panel like the one shown in Figure 8.5 would require the same punch-down tool as used to wire a single RJ45 socket – but there are some do's and don'ts that need to be adhered to, to avoid the cables becoming disordered or obstructive.

Figure 8.5   A patch panel

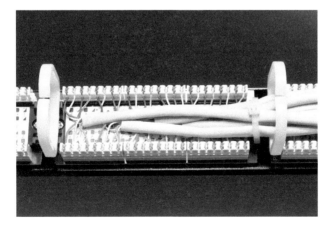

If not identified and prepared for, new variations or extensions of your core activities might leave you floundering on site, on what should have been an important day. Use the method statement template in Appendix D to help you identify these hurdles in advance.

Going forwards, try to favour suppliers who offer training or at least signposts to training. Purchasing takes up time, so look for suppliers who give something back.

With the patch panel example, there is training out there (with signposts provided to this in Appendix C), but would you have spotted that you needed it in time? Another reason to get in the habit of doing method statements is that they can help you spot gaps in advance.

8.8   The smart home HE

Location of the HE was discussed in Section 2.10.2.

The guidance in this Section suggests ways to make things easier when you come to assemble a well-featured HE – the centre-piece of your installation.

Smart home professionals like to put a lot of time and effort into perfecting this part of the installation. Publicizing good work in the form of a well-laid-out and tidy HE is encouraged.

8.8.1   The right enclosure

Figure 8.6 shows an example of the front of a purpose-built HE enclosure.

Figure 8.6   A smart home HE enclosure

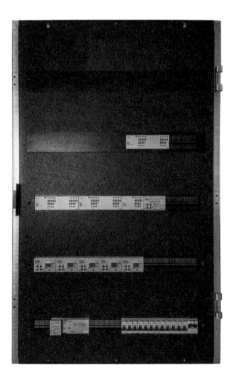

Most manufacturers design their modules to fit a DIN rail/letterbox format like a DB. You can buy, and stack, generic DIN rail/letter box enclosures, but be advised that that approach is unlikely to make it easy for you to achieve what you need to in terms of space and segregation in an HE. Something with plenty of space is preferable.

An experienced electrical installer will be able to build their own enclosure, starting with something along the lines of the enclosure shown in Figure 8.7, which comes in a variety of sizes.

Figure 8.7 An adaptable wall box

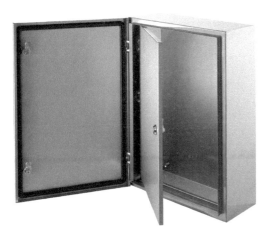

Before specifying an HE enclosure, ask your smart home manufacturer if they have an enclosure manufacturer they favour to house their modules. Some will have developed or co-developed their own to suit their configuration, and using that one might save you a lot of time and frustration. Buying a custom HE enclosure will save you having to source, assemble and position the accessories you are likely to need, as shown in Figure 8.8.

Figure 8.8 Example of a custom board

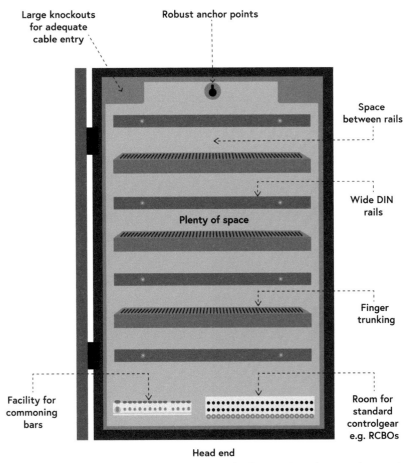

Note: Smart homes may have extra requirement for functional earthing, as discussed in Section 5.4. Ensure that there is adequate provision for earthing, bonding and protective conductor terminations within the HE.

8.8.2 The right terminals to make the right terminations

Running sheathed cables through your HE is a bad idea: you will run out of space quickly. Sheathed cables should be terminated close to the point of entry in a manner that makes them easy to wire onwards in the appropriate conductor, as shown in Figure 8.9.

Figure 8.9   Simplified illustration of bad (left) and good (right) termination strategies

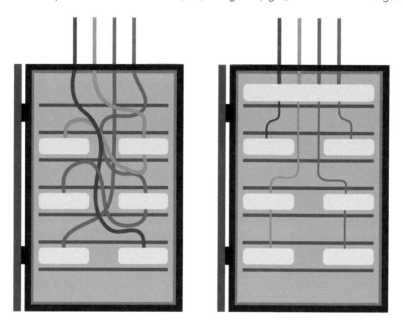

The cables on the right of Figure 8.9 would typically be run within finger trunking around the perimeter and along horizontal channels.

DIN connectors

Unfixed connectors like those shown in Figure 8.10 are not acceptable as a rule in an HE. Terminations and connections should be made in the appropriate DIN-mounted or suitably affixed connector.

Figure 8.10   Sub-standard wiring and connector

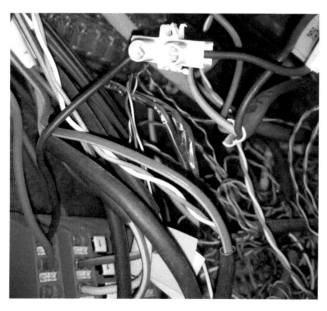

There are refinements of the classic in/out DIN connector on the market, which are better in terms of:

(a) handling thinner cores;
(b) ease of labelling;
(c) ease of connecting cables together (commoning);
(d) ease of insertion and removal; and
(e) space factor – they use less rail.

A variety of DIN connectors are shown in Figure 8.11.

Figure 8.11   In/out DIN connectors

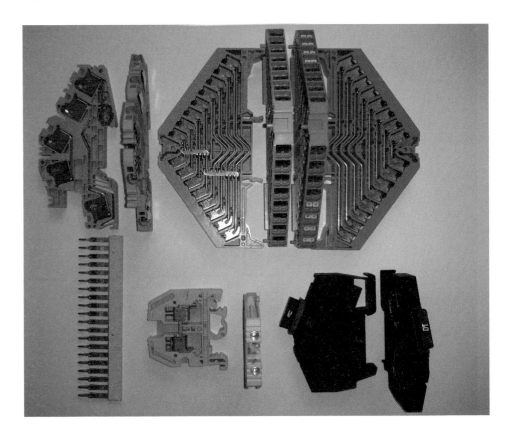

Where you do have to use a screw terminal for a single- or dual-core termination, the smart home industry expects you to use a bootlace ferrule, as shown on the left of Figure 8.12.

Ferrules are more robust and safer. Trouble-shooting in tight spaces is much easier if ferrules have been used.

Figure 8.12   Ferrule terminations next to a dangerous non-ferrule termination

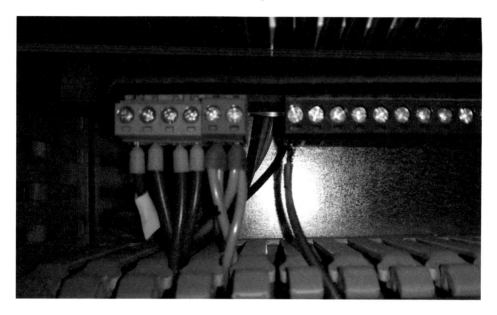

8.8.3 Plan your HE

Allow time to draw the layout and interconnections of your HE, ideally at the design stage, but definitely before you start installing. Proceed from the general, as in Figure 8.13, to the specific, as necessary.

Figure 8.13   An HE layout sketch

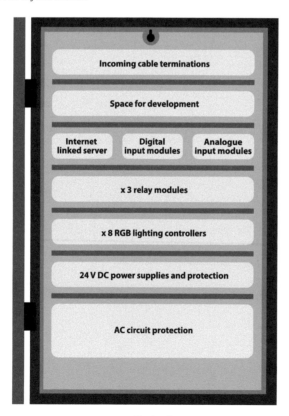

No matter how much time you spend designing your HE, it will be affected by errors and oversights. The finished product, however, will certainly be the better for your efforts.

An HE is not necessarily a single enclosure: it is a collection of whatever the smart home requires, grouped for convenience and functionality. A segmented HE is shown in Figure 8.14.

Things that an HE might incorporate include:

(a) low voltage AC (LVAC);
(b) low voltage DC (LVDC): battery energy storage and the possibility of renewable distributed LVDC energy;
(c) data/telecommunications: BT, Ethernet and protocols (for example, Modbus);
(d) ELVAC: for example, an alarm sounder;
(e) ELVDC: for example, LED lighting and device power; and
(f) AV.

Figure 8.14   An HE can be distributed

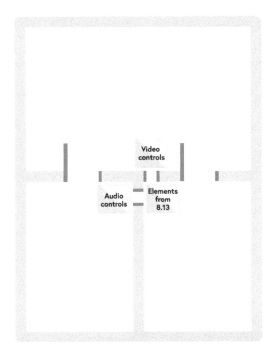

Zoning an enclosure

Your primary concern in designing and wiring the HE is ensuring that potentially lethal voltages are appropriately segregated from non-lethal voltage systems. This is business as usual for an electrical installer, but the extent of the proximity calls for extra attention.

Again, you should seek manufacturers' guidance. Ask them what you are likely to need that is outside the normal traditional scope, such as:

(a) specialist tools: for example, needle probes or punch down tools; and
(b) specialist protection: for example, DC fuses or thermal protection.

Can you arrange cables and components to make segregation easier?

Consider an enclosure like the one represented in Figure 8.15, with 24 V DC and 230 V AC within.

(a) Option A might require a bit of stud work in the ceiling to make 'letterboxes' for left/right cables;

(b) Option B might require a bit of boxing and extra cable to make it work; and

(c) Option C is easy to first fix, but will make your life very hard later on.

Figure 8.15   Enclosure with more than one energy class

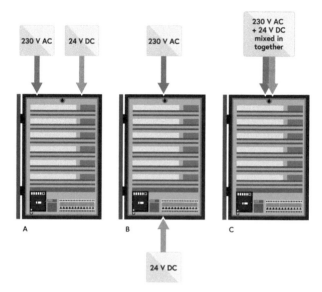

The best way to bring cables in will depend on the modules you have specified. Figure 8.16 shows a module that combines multiple energy classes. In fact, the eight relays on the bottom of the unit could each control a different energy class.

Figure 8.16   A typical module with I/Os labelled by energy class (Reproduced by permission of Loxone)

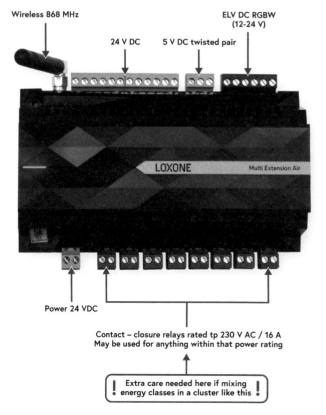

Diagrams like that in Figure 8.16 should be readily available from your smart home manufacturer. Can you see a way of arranging the modules to minimize congestion and proximity of different energy classes?

Consider printing the modules out and shuffling them around to find the best fit. When you think you have it, add the other things, such as DC power supplies and terminal blocks.

(a) Does it still fit?
(b) Do you need a bigger enclosure?
(c) Do you need a separate enclosure for power supplies, perhaps in another room?

Having answers to those questions in advance is very important.

Always seek manufacturers' guidance on considerations of layout. Few will want to design this for you, but all will have a list of known issues. For example, you might choose to put the whole house's circuit protection with RCD devices at the bottom or top of your HE – but this might cause interference which some devices will need separation from.

Separate enclosures

As you take on bigger smart home jobs, it is likely that you will need to specify HEs that need more than one enclosure. There is no right or wrong way to do this, so long as it is safe, and the system meets expectations.

Remember, though, that aesthetics are part of the client's expectations. Dinner guests for the next five years are likely to get a tour of the house that includes your HE. It should therefore reflect the planning, care and skill that the installer put into the whole job.

The following are suggestions to help you achieve a good result whilst you are learning.

As with the single-enclosure zoning example, consider using diagrams, cut-out paper or a CAD design tool to help you work out a good way to arrange equipment. By doing this in advance of the first fix, you can control where different cables emerge into the HE zone and minimize surface routing.

Where surface routing is required, plan for it and make it work for you. Consider incorporating trunking or ducting into your design. Size it so that it has scope for EMC segregation as described in Section 5.5 and for expansion when required. Figure 8.17 illustrates one such configuration.

Figure 8.17   Enclosure with trunking or ducting

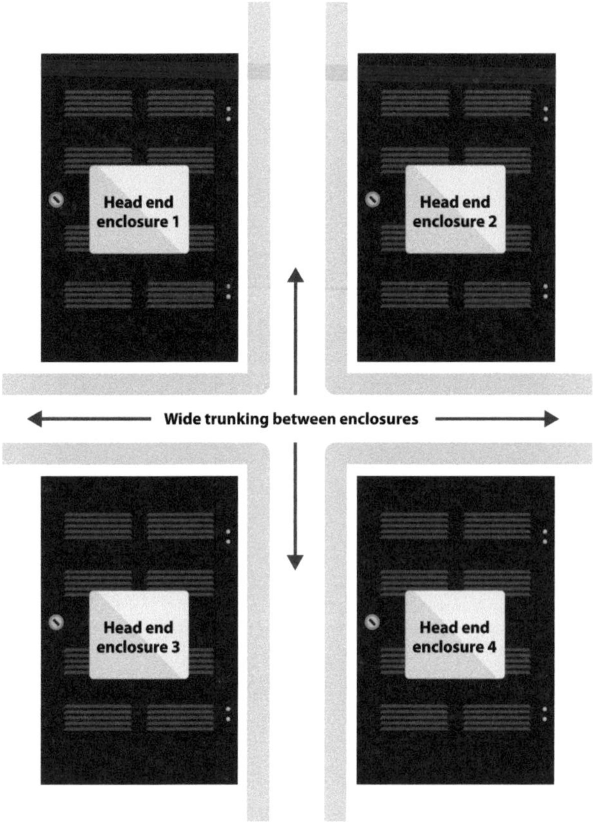

8.8.4   Enclosure compliance

Moving away from off-the-peg DB enclosures to custom assemblies requires attention to criteria for compliance, which include, but are not limited to, Regulation 421.1.201 of BS 7671:2018+A1:2020:

> *Within domestic (household) premises, consumer units and similar switchgear assemblies shall comply with BS EN 61439-3 and shall:*
> **(i)** *have their enclosure manufactured from non-combustible material, or*
> **(ii)** *be enclosed in a cabinet or enclosure constructed of non-combustible material and complying with Regulation 132.12.*

The combination of components from different manufacturers within the same enclosure is not best practice, but is often unavoidable for smart home systems. The potential issues are predominantly thermal; equipment that generates and can be detrimentally influenced by heat includes:

(a) lighting dimmers;
(b) power supplies;
(c) amplifiers; and
(d) controlgear.

Manufacturers' data sheets should contain information about heat generation and high-low temperature limits for operation.

The following measures are good practice:

(a) inclusion of a system-linked temperature sensor, which can trigger cooling measures and/or issue an alert. Always default to manufacturers' guidance, but as a rule of thumb, aim to maintain a temperature below 27 °C, with an alert at 35 °C. More guidance on environmental control for HE enclosures can be found in Section 4.3 of the IET *Code of Practice for Connected Systems Integration in Buildings*.

(b) where surge protection is used, include this within its own separate enclosure if the manufacturer's guidelines stipulate this.

(c) take precautions to avoid counterfeit components.

(d) size your enclosures to allow for air gaps between components: squeezing current-using components together acts in the same way as insulation, so give them air.

(e) consider arc-fault sensing measures.

Regulation 536.4.203 of BS 7671:2018+A1:2020 should be consulted when mixing components within an enclosure or a panel. Always seek manufacturers' guidance regarding compatibility.

8.9   Summary

A smart home project needs more active documentation and more diligence from start to finish:

(a) to safeguard the client, the end-user and the installer; and

(b) to provide for ease of operation and maintenance throughout its life.

The requirements will vary.

Try to stay on track with documentation and ensure that everything you do is documented in a way that could be easily and usefully included in the handover pack. If something you are doing is not documentable, take a step back and ask yourself why.

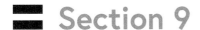 Section 9

How to commission a smart home system

This Section considers the steps required to effectively commission and hand over a smart home system to the end-user.

An experienced electrical installer knows the proper commissioning procedure for any electrical or electronic system:

(a) Inspection;
(b) Verification; and
(c) Testing:

leading to **C**ommissioning:

IVT → C

9.1 What is different for the electrical installer when commissioning a smart home?

For a smart home, the IVT of functional switching and controls involves working with more layers, including an IT layer. In addition, a smart home is likely to contain a greater variety of voltages.

This Section will help you to identify the best methodology for commissioning the system you have designed.

9.2 Inspection verification, and testing of fixed wiring and equipment to relevant standards

Where the system is complex and there are multiple members of an installation team, it is strongly recommended that the system designer leads the IVT. This should be the policy until all the challenges are quantified and planned for. Expecting any electrical installer to satisfactorily test a fully wired smart home without knowledge of how the system works is likely to lead to problems.

The inspection process is fundamentally unchanged, except that you may need to do it more times, due to more complex assembly.

Similarly, verification may need to be repeated more often, as additional control layers (for example, app-based devices) are added.

9.2.1   Testing mains voltage circuits

Until you are fully familiar with the smart home equipment, it is recommended that your default strategy for testing circuits (to the Installation Certificate schedules set out in BS 7671:2018+A1:2020) should be to link out or bypass electronic equipment, as illustrated in Figure 9.1.

Figure 9.1   Testing circuits

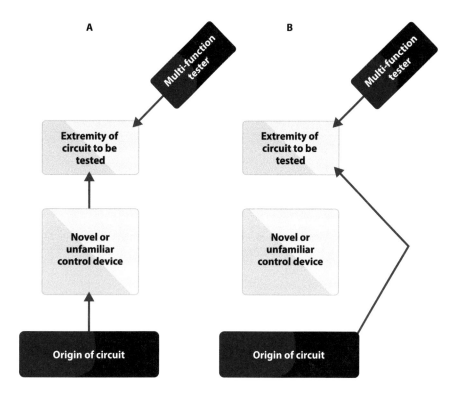

In Figure 9.1, the option B method has two advantages:

1   it eliminates the possibility that a false assumption about the connections within a sophisticated 'box' might lead to mistaken readings; and

2   it eliminates the possibility that you will damage electronic equipment with insulation resistance tests or, conceivably, loop impedance (Zs) tests.

A disadvantage is that you may spend more time testing – which isn't necessarily a negative thing. The multi-function tester should be on-site and in use during, and not just at the end of, any installation.

Building in time to test and verify as the installation proceeds might help you to spot an oversight. Recording the data will save you time when you come to complete your certificate.

Consideration will be needed as to what extent the circuit is fully verified if tests were conducted with control equipment bypassed. Disconnecting and bypassing current-using equipment is permitted in accordance with Regulation 643.3 of BS 7671:2018+A1:2020, but the outcome must ensure operational safety. Seek manufacturers' guidance if you are unsure.

9.2.2   LV and ELVDC power

Non-signal DC cabling – for example, lighting – should be tested for continuity, insulation resistance and polarity. These characteristics should be recorded. The suitability of the cables for the designated load should be confirmed in writing.

9.2.3 Ethernet

Specialist equipment is available to test Ethernet cables. Testers range from £5 for something that will speed up a continuity test to >£1,000 for something that will verify integrity and output a report. A smart home installer will initially have use for something in the middle, with the ability to detect cable length and distance to faults. Some models will incorporate adaptors for coaxial cable and phone as well.

Figure 9.2   Ethernet testers

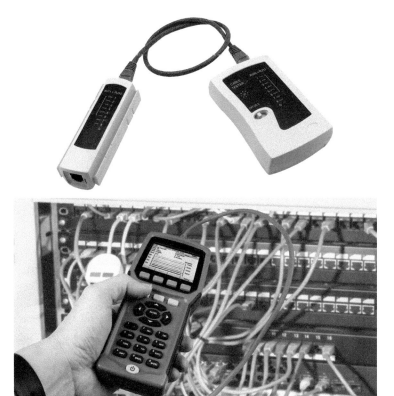

9.2.4 Other signal cables

Follow manufacturers' guidelines where available, and as a minimum, always verify continuity and insulation resistance.

9.3   Functional commissioning

With fixed wiring testing complete, you can proceed to commissioning for functionality. This should be carried out by comparison with the functional analysis that was prepared at the design stage and included with the proposal.

9.3.1 Configuration

Obviously, it is impossible to complete commissioning until someone has programmed – or as it is more commonly termed, 'configured' – the system. Therefore, it is wise to plan for that requirement.

The amount of configuration required will depend on the product. The preparation required to configure competently should have been established with the manufacturer during the design stage.

Where configuration is likely to be extensive, consider doing the configuration off-site in advance of commissioning. For more straightforward systems, particularly IoT systems for which the commissioning is based on the client's network, this will not be an option, as the programming will all be done via the local router.

Refer to the manufacturers' guidance on best procedure for commissioning. For some products, this will be on the literature in the box, under a heading like 'set-up'. More advanced systems should have step-by-step guidance on how to commission efficiently. Some will have features within the UI or configuration software to help you complete commissioning.

Have a system for naming files so that you can easily track changes. Include the date and time and some memory aid as to what you just did: for example, "2017 04 15 incorporated landing PIR into intruder alarm 1425". This simple step can save you a lot of frustration if you have to subsequently trouble-shoot.

9.3.2 Functional commissioning procedure

Each installation will be different, but the following procedure can be used as a guide:

(a) consider this as a rehearsal for the handover;
(b) go through the functional analysis as if the client were with you;
(c) tick off features as you progress through zones testing them;
(d) be methodical and record glitches before you detour to fix them; and
(e) keep a record of all remedial actions taken, for both software and hardware.

The criteria for the proper commissioning of a smart home are as follows:

(a) have all the relevant standards, including, but not limited to BS 7671:2018+A1:2020, been met?
(b) have all reasonable considerations and precautions been taken to ensure the operational safety of the system? (It is possible to have an electrically compliant device that can lead to injury or misfortune.)
(c) Have the client's expectations been met?

Remember: a good commissioning procedure, referencing a good functional analysis, is a great alternative to a snag list.

9.4 Commissioning documentation

In addition to mandatory certification and certificates, it is recommended that you create a diagram and/or a schedule of the following:

(a) the circuit protection layout, explained in Section 9.4.1;
(b) the HE internal layout, explained in Section 9.4.2; and
(c) the HE external layout, explained in Section 9.4.3.

9.4.1 Circuit protection layout

The traditional circuit schedule, as found on a BS 7671 Electrical Installation Certificate, might not be sufficient to capture the detail of how circuit-breakers relate to final circuits.

Consider the arrangement shown in Figure 9.3. A single MCB feeds one relay module, which in turn serves 12 final circuits spanning multiple functional classes.

Section 9 – How to commission a smart home system

Figure 9.3   MCB feeding relays on a module

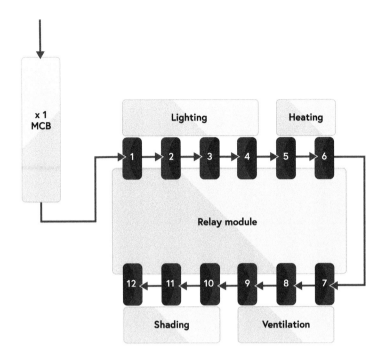

You should have a means of recording how a given MCB way relates to final circuits in the installation. The grouping can be very different to a traditional installation. A template for recording final circuits downstream of an MCB way can be found in Appendix D. The requirements of Regulation 514.9 (Diagrams and documentation) of BS 7671:2018+A1:2020 should be adhered to.

Figure 9.4 presents one-way information about how circuit protection might be organized. The detail required will vary with the complexity of the installation.

Figure 9.4   Example of circuit protection layout

Protective device	Location	Neutral termination	Line termination	Intermediate terminations	Module termination	Final circuits
6 A RCBO 30 mA	DB1 way 4	HE neutral bar #6	Relay module 4 digital output 1–8	NA	NA	Shading beds 1–4
						Central heating boiler call
						Landing pendant luminaire
						Cloakroom extractor fan
						Kitchen tea towel radiator
16 A RCBO 30 mA	DB1 way 5	SHHE neutral bar #7	Relay module 6 digital output 2		NA	Immersion element hot water tank
6 A RCBO 30 mA	DB1 way 6	24 V DC PSU (100 W) #1	24 V DC PSU #1	x2 8-way DIN connectors Top rail #7 /#12 +ve	DMX controller #3	Bathroom RGB LED strip
					NA	Window closure contacts ground floor

9.4.2 HE internal layout

Where you have created and wired an HE, as shown in Figure 9.5, you should also create something like the terminal map shown in Figure 9.6.

Figure 9.5   Well-featured HE

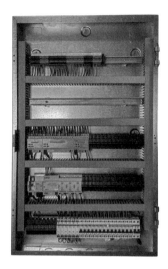

Figure 9.6   A map of terminals (Reproduced by permission of CEDIA)

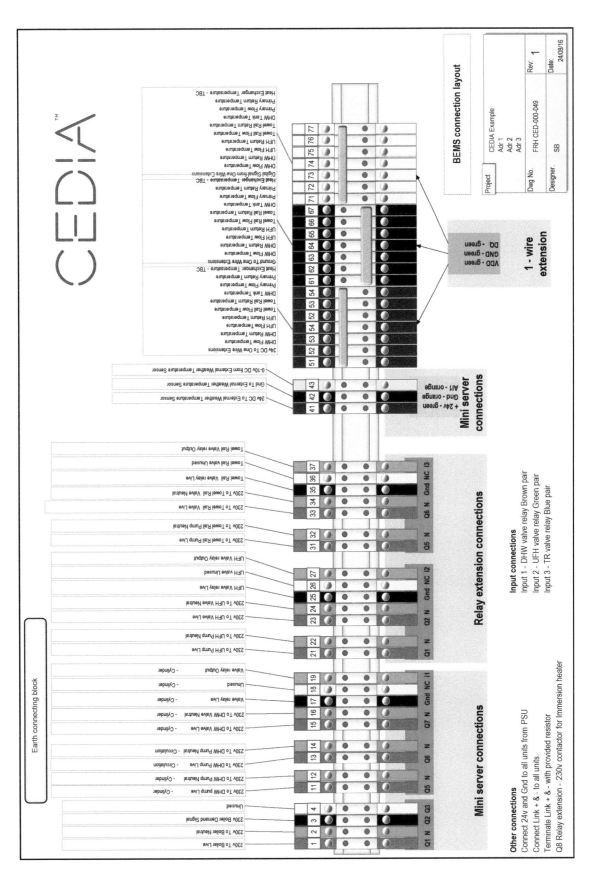

The precise layout and detail will vary with the equipment and project. Where a graphical representation is not possible, the minimum requirement is for all terminals to be numbered and for a list of circuits corresponding to numbers to be shown.

A similar illustration for structured cabling for a patch panel is shown in Figure 9.7.

Figure 9.7   Ethernet patch panel map (Reproduced by permission of CEDIA)

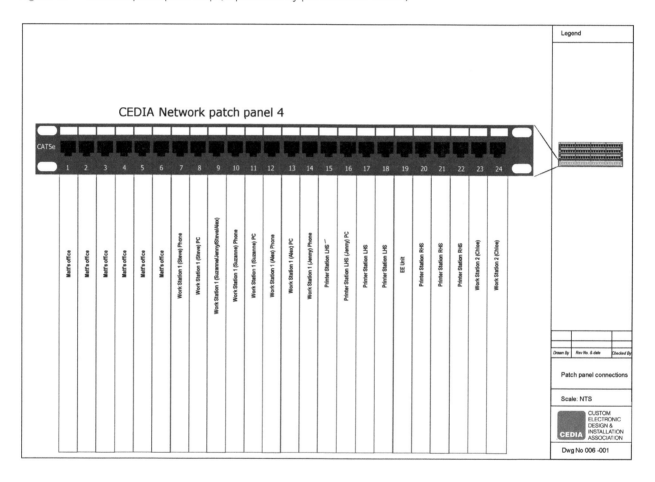

9.4.3   HE external layout

Every input, output and control must be clearly and permanently labelled. It is not enough to label the cable or patch lead connected to it.

Where space does not permit for a descriptive label, use a code that can be referenced to a separate schedule.

9.5   Commissioning summary

Think of your commissioning procedure as a last inspection before you (in your imagination, at least) move on to another job in another country.

Set up all hardware, software and documentation so that another appropriately skilled technician could come to the job and make sense of what you have done.

Leaving labelled cores for following trades can save you an unpaid call-out: for example, the shades might be supplied by a third party long after you have finished your work, and if the cores in the outlet are properly labelled, they might not need you to be there.

You created this system and you should be the one who supports it. We will review the documentation that you have generated in Section 9.8. If done well, it will reflect your professionalism and you will be the one who benefits from it, as you will then be able to carry out lucrative maintenance and referrals.

9.6 Handover

The components and controls of smart homes are still immature and unfamiliar technology compared with traditional electrical homes. Many clients will struggle to understand or operate their new smart home or in-home smart device without your help.

Neglecting handover will unravel all of your good smart home work so far, at least in the client's eyes.

The software configuration is the core of the handover. It is as much a part of what the client paid for as the hardware, and it is their property.

You must leave the client with everything they need to benefit from and enjoy using the system you have installed.

Refer back to the two broad categories of smart home applications described in Section 1.5:

1. smart home lifestyle products (note that lifestyle can be a symptom of physical circumstances, such as a disability); and
2. smart home energy management products.

Do not neglect either category – and weight the delivery of the handover to match the installation. Where the installation is lifestyle-led, explanation will be a natural process.

With energy-management considerations, explanation may need to be more structured, but it should not be neglected. The users' understanding of the system will help them to optimize savings.

Additionally, as an electrical installer, you have a mandate to deliver buildings that comply with forward-thinking sustainability regulations, including, but not limited to, those set out here:

> Approved Document Part L1A: *Conservation of fuel and power* of the Building Regulations:
>
> Criterion 5 – Provisions for energy-efficient operation of the dwelling
>
> 4.1 In accordance with regulation 40, the owner of the dwelling should be provided with sufficient information about the building, the fixed building services and their maintenance requirements so that the building can be operated in such a manner as to use no more fuel and power than is reasonable in the circumstances.
>
> 4.3 b. Explain how to operate, control and maintain the following systems:
>
>   i. space heating system;
>   ii. hot water heating system;
>   iii. ventilation system;
>   iv. any other technology which has been included in the dwelling, e.g. solar panels or other low and zero carbon technology, or a technology for which SAP Appendix Q has been utilized.

9.7   The shape of a good handover

The handover for each installation will be different. The following can be used as a guide.

(a) Plan for handover all the way through and include it in the costing.
(b) Match the extent of the handover to the complexity of the installation.
(c) Allow enough time for the handover, as rushing it is as bad as omitting it. For a fully featured five-bed smart home, allow half a day to take clients through it and deal with questions (there may be a lot of them).
(d) Encourage the householder to think of your handover pack as the central resource to the installation.

9.8   Handover pack documentation

The handover pack could include:

(a) cable schedules.
(b) diagrams or schedules of inputs, outputs and significant components within the HE.
(c) cable schematics, where practical.

Note: Items (a)–(c) are things that you created at the design stage which might have been altered during installation and commissioning. Aim to create and maintain documents to a standard where they can be handed over with a minimum of work. Having to produce a new version of everything, if you neglect to keep documents in good order, will be onerous.

(d) electrical certificates, typically BS 7671 Electrical Installation Certificates.
(e) other diagrams/notices/schedules as appropriate, or as required by BS 7671:2018+A1:2020 or any other relevant standards. Examples include:
   (i) your diagrams/schedules of the MCB way to final circuits;
   (ii) electromagnetic 'heat mapping' certificates;
   (iii) structured cabling performance certificates;
   (iv) acoustic performance certificates; and
   (v) notification for building installations – this may arrive later, but leave a clear space for it in your pack.
(f) product documentation.

Note: This can be digital or hard-copy. Remember that your aim is to create a user manual for the house, so a simple list of links to manufacturers' websites is not helpful. Similarly, a device's 140-page instruction book in nine languages will make your pack impressively thick – but again, is not helpful. Filter content to make your handover pack genuinely useful.

(g) bespoke instructions.

Note: User-information provided by manufacturers may not be fit for purpose. Create resources the householder can refer to after you have moved on from the job and the memory of your excellent handover has faded.

Basic trouble-shooting could be covered: for example, a reminder for people to check if their internet is working before they call you due to a perceived failure. Similarly, you might want to leave guidance on how to change batteries, as shown in Figure 9.8.

Figure 9.8   Example instructions

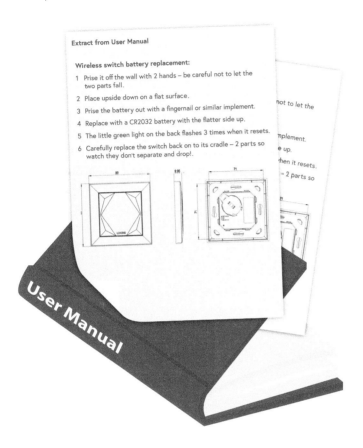

Extract from User Manual

Wireless switch battery replacement:

1 Prise it off the wall with 2 hands – be careful not to let the two parts fall.

2 Place upside down on a flat surface.

3 Prise the battery out with a fingernail or similar implement.

4 Replace with a CR2032 battery with the flatter side up.

5 The little green light on the back flashes 3 times when it resets.

6 Carefully replace the switch back on to its cradle – 2 parts so watch they don't separate and drop!.

(h) software and cyber-security elements. Include:

(i) a copy of the configuration software, as demonstrated at the handover, on solid-state, cloud storage or by email.

(ii) a notice of client usernames and passwords, with instructions to change at least the passwords. The supporting technician should take steps to safeguard their own username and password, subject to permission and the GDPR guidelines.

(iii) a summary of any software or cyber-security requirements of the job.

(i) a copy of the functional analysis from your commissioning procedure.

Note: Items from the functional analysis should be ticked off as they are demonstrated.

(j) confirmation of completion of handover.

Note: This is to be signed by the installer and the householder when all the items on the functional analysis are completed and questions have been dealt with. Consider having a field for a witness signature. An example template of how a functional analysis can be adapted with a column for a handover tick list can be found in Appendix D.

(k) a maintenance schedule, including an itemization of actions to be carried out to ensure the safe and effective operation of the system, with recommended intervals.

Note: This should have been referred to in your contract or agreement. You might choose to offer a support contract for consideration at this point.

9.9 Conducting the handover

Manage expectations: make sure in advance that the householder understands what needs to happen and that all parties concerned have the time to do it properly.

Structure the delivery: don't bombard the client with verbal information or with every detail of your manual.

Walk and talk, show and tell. Room by room, demonstrate features, and then allow the client time to try these out through the variety of controls configured for phone, tablet or wall button, as they prefer. Tick off features on the functional analysis as you go.

Safety critical features and considerations should be given emphasis by the electrical installer in the handover.

Demonstrate how to perform simple manual tasks such as isolating equipment or changing a battery in a wireless device. Leave a set of spare batteries identified by device in the handover pack, with some indication of battery life expectation. This is the sort of proactive behaviour that can win hearts and save you a call-out.

Let the client have a look through the manual you have created for them at the end. Allow time for questions arising from the manual.

Explain where you have briefed other contractors how to operate the system for functional checks. For example, swimming pool installers might need to know more than the client about certain aspects of your pump control system.

When all reasonable questions have been answered, you are clear to have any outstanding paperwork signed.

9.10 Handover summary

Of course, your relationship with the installation and the householder does not stop there. You have the same obligations and responsibilities as a smart home contractor as you would for a traditional installation.

A good handover of a good installation brings the following benefits:

(a) a happy customer;
(b) fewer follow-up issues caused by misunderstandings;
(c) opportunity for ongoing support work; and
(d) referrals to further interesting projects.

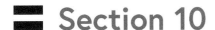 **Section 10**

Supporting the smart home

This Section considers the additional opportunities and challenges involved with the continued support of a smart home installation.

10.1 What is different for the electrical installer supporting smart homes?

A secure and compliant standard installation is likely to need minimal support and maintenance. For a smart home, there will be an opportunity for more follow-up:

(a) smart systems need IT maintenance;

(b) IT support might be provided remotely;

(c) IT support might be provided out of office hours; and

(d) smart home maintenance contracts offer a greater revenue opportunity than traditional installations.

Specific support elements will vary between installations.

Consider that if you don't provide support, someone else will certainly have to – probably a competitor, who will be only too happy to improve on your work and handle referrals for you.

Being effective in a support role will require more than just answering the phone and turning up when there is a problem. Client-facing support is what electrical installers are used to and geared up for, and while this is still present, there is a further dimension to smart home support.

10.2 Industry-facing support obligations

In Section 1.3.1 we mentioned the requirement for a sincere and sustained interest to be a useful part of the smart home industry. Offering support for a smart home installation will require significant industry-facing activity on the part of the installer. This industry is constantly moving and developing, and the smart home installer needs to keep up.

Examples of industry-facing activities which become your responsibility are considered below.

10.2.1 Monitoring manufacturer developments

Known issues

Manufacturers aren't likely to publish a list of things that don't work as they should with their products. They should, however, let their partners know about issues likely to affect satisfaction and safety. Make sure you are subscribed to this information channel and have the capacity to act on it.

Software updates

As with known issues, make sure you are alerted to software updates, preferably in advance, so that you can schedule activities such as firmware updates.

Each update should come with a changelog detailing what has been changed. You must read and consider this. Does it address any issues you or your clients have encountered? Should you adjust any of your configurations to take advantage of improvements?

Section 10 – Supporting the smart home

Additions or improvements to devices

Keep your eyes open for devices that improve what you can offer to your clients.

Telling people about an amazing new version of something they bought only last month can lead to tension, however, so tact is required. Nevertheless, where there is a technology development that can offer the client a better experience, it is your responsibility to let them know about it.

Training

You have an ethical obligation to maintain your knowledge and skills so that you can keep the systems you have supplied optimized. Keep abreast of developments and available training. You should have assessed the requirements and costs associated with this before specifying a particular manufacturer's equipment.

10.2.2 Monitoring wider industry developments

People will be spending money to incorporate infrastructure based on your recommendations. As a trusted smart home practitioner, you cannot blindly rely on just one manufacturer forever.

Make time, therefore, to review new technological possibilities, which fall broadly into two categories:

1. new devices from smart manufacturers; and
2. new possibilities for integrating periphery systems with smart devices.

10.3 Client-facing support opportunities

10.3.1 On-site maintenance

A schedule for on-site maintenance should have been included in the handover pack.

Your activities are likely to focus at the HE: attention to distributed devices will probably be on a sample or response-to-issue basis.

An example of scheduled activities might include the following:

(a) issuing a BS 7671 Electrical Installation Condition Report (EICR) and meeting equivalent requirements.
(b) assessing the physical integrity of the enclosures and the components within.
(c) assessing the physical integrity of the electrical connections (the use of thermal imaging is strongly recommended in an HE where there are numerous connections).
(d) checking ventilation is functioning and is not obstructed by dust or objects.
(e) carrying out a product-specific inspection. Consult manufacturers' guidelines with respect to inspection requirements for the equipment you have supplied.
(f) carrying out a peripheral item inspection. For equipment you did not supply, but which is controlled by the system you installed, it is desirable to inspect in line with manufacturers' guidance and to anticipate problems. It is recommended that you keep photographic records.

10.3.2 Preparing for on-site maintenance

Give yourself a chance to be prepared. Communicate with the client in advance: find out if anyone in the household is having any issues or if there are any additions or adjustments required. If this is the case, you may have to:

(a) go to site with parts or tools you might not otherwise have expected to need;

(b) reschedule; or

(c) consult or bring in third parties.

10.3.3 Remote maintenance

Remote maintenance caution

While all the support activities might be performed remotely via an internet connection, you should proceed with caution at the start in this respect. Unforeseen issues can arise from alterations to configuration and it is therefore advisable to be on-site where possible for the first round of changes. Do not be tempted to earn money by doing IT maintenance whilst on holiday – unless you have a contingency plan should things go awry. Wait at least until you have a dozen such installations under your belt.

Software updates

IT support requirements will vary between installations. The following points may serve as a guide:

(a) within a specific scope, agreed as per the GDPR, you may access devices directly or via the LAN to update software on the system or devices;

(b) many systems will be able to update remotely;

(c) while auto-updating might be the norm for screen-based apps, it is not the norm for smart home systems;

(d) the safest option is to conduct updates whilst on-site, in case issues arise; and

(e) consult the manufacturer to see what they advise.

System health checks

Within a specific scope, agreed as per the GDPR, you may access devices directly or via the LAN to check that the system is functioning normally. This could include checking that:

(a) all components are communicating;

(b) memory caches are not full; and

(c) the UI is as it should be.

System optimization

By agreement, you might adjust the configuration to take advantage of software updates or in the light of system performance data.

10.4 How to record support and maintenance

All support and maintenance activities should be logged. This should be done in a consistent, agreed format, and it makes sense to follow the format of the handover pack. If this was digital, then your support and maintenance documentation should be digital. If it was a hard copy, then your folder should have an identifiable section for inclusion of support and maintenance reports. The exact content of the support and maintenance report will depend on the job and should be compiled based on manufacturer guidelines.

10.4.1 Ad hoc support

Have a system for logging written and verbal conversations. With email, it is very easy to frame the initial request or query with your response. Where communication is verbal, you should still record particulars of the conversation, including the date, time and subject against the actions you took.

This might seem like overkill, but consider that you might assume that a configuration adjustment is appropriate, and make three more changes, before you realise it was in fact a hardware issue. Have you recorded your configuration changes and the reason they were made?

A summary of all ad hoc support issues should be made available for inclusion within the smart home pack.

10.5 Summary of the smart home support opportunity

Sections 10.2–10.4 are an outline of what is required for offering support for smart homes and smart home devices. Only the designer can really say what support is necessary for a given system.

Bear in mind that you cannot charge for industry-facing elements directly. You will have to think carefully about how to structure and price the client-facing elements to make them viable.

If you can do all of this well, there is real potential for good, lucrative work. However, you might need to consider new business strategies to ensure that a support system is in place.

Be creative and prepared to think 'out of the box'. Perhaps it is a good idea to create some sort of partnership with someone who will take on all the responsibility for support? There are already businesses that offer this as a service. They will have their own requirements and terms, which you should research thoroughly before making any sort of commitment.

In any event, approach the smart home revolution with an open mind to opportunity and an awareness of risk. With good planning and care, the two can be balanced to produce exciting prospects and better buildings.

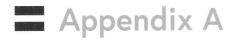

Appendix A

Abbreviations and glossary

Term	Definition
AC	*alternating current* An electric current flowing in both directions along a conductor successively
Administrator	A system operator with access to all settings
ADS	*automatic disconnection of supply* An arrangement of circuit protection including earthing, where electrical faults will cause the faulty circuit to be disconnected from the supply
AI	*artificial intelligence* A system able to perform tasks normally requiring human intelligence. Also called *machine learning*
AP	*access point (WiFi)* A device that effectively provides an antenna for a router
API	*application programming interface* A set of functions and procedures allowing the creation of applications that access the features or data of an operating system, application or other service
Applet	A very small application, especially a utility programme performing one or a few simple functions
Architecture	The design of a given object or system
Assisted Living	The application of technology to make life easier for those with mobility or other challenges
AV	*audiovisual*
BACS	*building automation and control systems*
Balun	A device to provide impedance transformation between balanced and unbalanced components
BEF	*building entrance facility* A physical location where services enter a structure
BOM	*bill of materials* A list of materials used in a project
Bonding	A protective conductor providing equipotential bonding
BUS	*bus network* A bus network is an arrangement in a local area network (*LAN*) in which each node (workstation or other device) is connected to a main cable or link called the 'bus'
Cache	Reserved areas of memory in a system that are used to speed up processing
CAD	*computer-aided design*
CAT cable	A twisted pair cable for computer and extra-low voltage (*ELV*) communication networks. Most commonly with 4-twisted pairs
CCTV	*closed-circuit television*
CDM	*Construction (Design and Management) Regulations* This is a set of Regulations that apply to every construction project in Great Britain
Cloud server/storage/computing	The practice of using a network of remote servers hosted on the internet to store, manage and process data, rather than a local server or a personal computer
CMS	*cable management system* A structure that physically supports or contains cables and conductors
Commissioning	The process of assuring that all systems and components of the smart home are operationally safe and in accordance with the client's expectations
Compatibility	The ability of one device or piece of software to work with another
Consumer tech	Smart home devices that can be purchased from general retail, which do not necessarily require specialist skills to install or operate
CPR	*Construction Product Regulation* Harmonized rules for construction products in the EU
CSA	*cross-sectional area*
DB	*distribution board* Also referred to as consumer units. A node that is usually an enclosure, where electrical current is split into separate circuits which each have overcurrent protection appropriate to their application
DC	*direct current* An electric current flowing in one direction only
Earthing	Measures taken to connect an electrical installation to the general mass of Earth. In the context of domestic installations, this will be to ensure that automatic disconnection of supply (*ADS*) can take place in the event of a fault
EES	*electric energy storage* A device that stores electrical energy for later use
ELV	*extra-low voltage* Not exceeding 50 V AC or 120 V ripple-free DC, whether between conductors or to earth
ELVDC	*extra-low voltage direct current*

Appendix A – Abbreviations and glossary

Term	Definition
ELVHE	*extra-low voltage head end*
EM	*electromagnetic*
EMC	*electromagnetic compatibility* The extent to which systems are able to operate properly adjacent to one another
EMI	*electromagnetic interference* Degradation of the performance of equipment, a transmission channel or a system caused by an electromagnetic disturbance
EMR	*electromagnetic radiation*
Energy mesh	A group of electrical loads configured to optimize a resource such as natural light or on-site microgeneration
EoP	*Ethernet over Power* An arrangement of devices that allows Ethernet signals to be transmitted over low-voltage (230 V AC) cables
Ethernet	A system for connecting a number of computer systems to form a local area network (*LAN*), with protocols to control the passing of information and to prevent simultaneous transmission by two or more systems
EU	*European Union*
EV	*electric vehicle*
Future-readying	The principle or practice of designing places and systems so that future developments can be incorporated at a later date
GDPR	*General Data Protection Regulation* A Regulation by which the European Parliament, the Council of the European Union and the European Commission intend to strengthen and unify data protection for all individuals within the European Union (*EU*)
Geo-mapping	The use of a global positioning system (GPS) or other locational technology to inform smart home system operation
HAN	*home area network* A type of computer network that facilitates communication among devices within the close vicinity of a home
Handover	A procedure where the smart home installer introduces the householder to the system and its supporting materials after proper commissioning
HBES	*home and building electronic system* An alternative term to smart home system
HE	*head end* A physical or virtual zone where smart home control is centralized
HEM	*home energy management* A measure that refines the conservation of energy in a building
Hub	A device at the centre of a number of devices that provides interconnection
ICT	*information and communications technology*
IFTTT	*If This Then That* A free web-based service to create chains of simple conditional statements, called applets
Interoperability	The ability of equipment or equipment groups to operate in conjunction with each other
IoT	*Internet of Things* The interconnection, via the internet, of computing devices embedded in everyday objects, enabling them to send and receive data
IP	*internet protocol* An addressing system for the internet
IT	*information technology* The study or use of systems (especially computers and telecommunications) for storing, retrieving and sending information
KNX	A well-established open standard for commercial and domestic building automation. Manufacturers and installers can be members of this organization
LAN	*local area network* (As *HAN*)
Layer	A term used to distinguish groups of functions within a network. The physical layer is at the bottom and the user interface (*UI*) is at the top
Light-harvesting	Any measure designed to use natural light instead of artificial light
LV	*low voltage* Exceeding extra-low voltage (*ELV*) but not exceeding 1,000 V AC or 1,500 V DC between conductors, or 600 V AC or 900 V DC between conductors and earth
LVDC	*low voltage DC*
Machine learning	See *AI*
M-Bus	A European standard for the remote reading of water, gas or electricity meters

Term	Definition
MEC	*main earthing conductor* A conductor connecting the main earthing terminal (*MET*) to the installation's means of earthing; for example, an earth rod
Mesh-network	A type of network that has no set path or route for communication. Each node can act as a transmitter or receiver to any adjacent node
MET	*main earthing terminal* The terminal or bar provided for the connection of protective conductors, including protective bonding conductors, and conductors for functional earthing, if any, to the means of earthing
MVHR	*mechanical ventilation heat recovery* A system that processes air to maintain quality and conserve heat
Needs analysis	Also referred to as a 'requirement analysis'. A process whereby the smart home designer gathers information from the householder about how they live and what they need from their home
OLEV	*Office for Low Emission Vehicles* A government organization responsible for implementing systems to facilitate the adoption of energy-efficient vehicles
Open source/shared source	Software that has been made available to developers or end-users. Terms and conditions vary
OS	*operating system* Software that manages computer hardware and software resources and provides common services for computer programmes
OSI	*open systems interconnection* A conceptual model that characterizes and standardizes the communication functions of a telecommunications or computing system without regard to its underlying internal structure and technology
PAS	*publicly available specification* A document that standardizes elements of a product, service or process. PASs are usually commissioned by industry leaders, such as individual companies, small and medium-sized enterprises (SMEs), trade associations and government departments
PC	*principal contractor* In the CDM, the party responsible for carrying out the work
PD	*principal designer* In the CDM, the party responsible for the design of the work
PE	*protective (Earth) conductor* A conductor intended to provide a fault path that can allow for *ADS* to occur
PELV	*protective extra-low voltage* An *ELV* system that is not electrically separated from Earth, but which otherwise satisfies all the requirements for *SELV*
PEN	*phase earth neutral* A conductor combining the functions of both a protective conductor and a neutral conductor
Platform	An environment in which software or services operate
PLC	*power-line communication* A standard for delivering *EoP*
Plug and play	A standard for the connection of devices to wider networks, where a simple unskilled operation enables operation
PoE	*Power over Ethernet* An arrangement of devices that allows *ELVDC* power to be transmitted through Ethernet cables. It utilizes the two twisted pairs in the Ethernet cable that are not required for standard networking
Protocol	Any combination of physical and software elements that provides a means of communication between devices
PV	*photovoltaics* Technology that converts light into electrical energy
Raspberry Pi	A series of small, single-board computers developed to promote the teaching of basic computer science
Router	A networking device that forwards data packets between computer networks. Usually found connected to the incoming telephone master socket
RP	*remote powering* Delivery of power to a device using the cable elements of information technology (*IT*) cable
SCS	*safety critical systems* Concerning any system the failure or malfunction of which may result in one (or more) of the following outcomes: (a) death or serious injury to people; (b) loss or severe damage to equipment or property; or (c) environmental harm
Segregation	Use of earthed, electrically conductive barriers or physical separation to prevent *EMI* between external noise sources, including power supply cabling and information technology (*IT*) cabling

Appendix A – Abbreviations and glossary

Term	Definition
SELV	*separated extra-low voltage* An *ELV* system that is electrically separated from Earth and from other systems in such a way that a single fault cannot give rise to the risk of electric shock
Server	A system that responds to requests across a computer network worldwide to provide, or help to provide, a network or data service
SETS	*smart electrical thermal storage* Any appliance that stores and releases thermal energy timed to achieve a strategic or financial advantage
SHHE	*smart home head end* Also referred to as the HE. The point to which all monitored and controlled devices are connected back
Smart device	Any device that delivers a smart measure
Smart home	A home that incorporates smart measures. Typically containing layers of technology between the user and the things that are controlled
Smart measure	Any arrangement that uses technology to facilitate better outcomes
SPD	*surge protection device* A device intended to protect electrical apparatus from high transient over-voltages and to limit the duration and frequently the amplitude of the follow-on current
Structured cabling	The design and installation of a cabling system that will support multiple hardware uses and be suitable for today's needs and those of the future. Typically made up of Ethernet cable and accessories
System integrators	Technicians with the competencies required to make different manufacturers' systems and different types of systems work together
TCP/IP	*transmission control protocol/internet protocol* A suite of communication protocols used to interconnect network devices on the internet or on a private computer network
TOU	*time of use tariff* A tariff for electricity in which the price per unit is dependent on when the electricity is used
Topography	The spatial arrangement of the physical features of an area
Topology	The way in which constituent parts of a system or environment are connected
UFH	*underfloor heating* An arrangement where a heat emitter is set into the floor
UPS	*uninterruptible power supply* A system that will provide a degree of power instantaneously in the event of a power cut
USB	*universal serial bus* A standard for cables and connectors and protocols for connection, communication and power supply between electronic devices
UI	*user interface* Any device that a user directly operates to control or monitor systems
V2G	*Vehicle-to-grid* An arrangement where electrical energy can be transferred in either direction between an electric vehicle (*EV*) and the grid
V2H	*Vehicle-to-home* An arrangement where electrical energy can be transferred in either direction between an electric vehicle and the home
WiFi	A family of wireless networking technologies, based on the IEEE 802.11 family of Standards

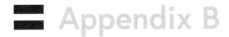

Appendix B

References

BSI (2016). BS EN 6701:2016+A1:2017 *Telecommunications equipment and telecommunications cabling. Specification for installation, operation and maintenance*. London: BSI.

BSI (2018). BS 7671:2018+A1:2020 *Requirements for Electrical Installations. IET Wiring Regulations*. London: BSI and the IET.

Department for Energy, Business and Industrial Strategy (2017). *Clean Growth Strategy*. [pdf] (Last updated 16 April 2018). Available at: https://www.gov.uk/government/publications/clean-growth-strategy

> *The Clean Growth Strategy identifies the key enablers and requirements of the shift to low-carbon transport and a low-carbon economy*

EU Publications Office (2010). *Directive 2010/31/EU of the European Parliament and of the Council of 19 May 2010 on the energy performance of buildings (EPBD)*. [online] (Last reviewed 8 August 2018). Available at: https://eur-lex.europa.eu/legal-content/EN/ALL/;ELX_SESSIONID=FZMjThLLzfxmmMCQG p2Y1s2d3TjwtD8QS3pqdkhXZbwqGwlgY9KN!2064651424?uri=CELEX:32010L0031

IET (2016). *Code of Practice for Connected Systems Integration in Buildings*. London: IET Standards.

BS EN 50174-2:2018 *Information technology. Cabling installation. Installation planning and practices inside buildings* (as referenced by BS 7671:2018+A1:2020)

Approved Document Part L: *Conservation of fuel and power*

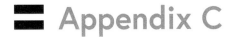 # Appendix C

Suggested further reading and resources

Systems integration and telecommunications cabling

ANSI/CEA/CEDIA/InfoComm (2015). ANSI-J-STD-710 *Audio, Video and Control Architectural Drawing Symbols Standard* (CEA/CEDIA-2039)

BSI (2015). PD CLC/TR 50174-99-1:2015 *Information technology. Cabling installation. Remote powering.* London: BSI.

BSI (2016). BS EN 6701:2016+A1:2017: *Telecommunications equipment and telecommunications cabling Specification for installation, operation and maintenance.* London: BSI.

BSI (2017). PAS 35491:2017 *Design and installation of telecommunications and broadcast infrastructure within the home. Code of practice.* London: BSI.

BSI (2018). BS EN 50173-1:2018 *Information technology. Generic cabling systems. General requirements.* London: BSI.

BSI (2018). BS EN 50173-4:2018 *Information technology. Generic cabling systems. Homes.* London: BSI.

BSI (2018). BS EN 50174-1:2018 *Information technology. Cabling installation. Installation specification and quality assurance.* London: BSI.

BSI (2018). BS EN 50174-2:2018 *Information technology. Cabling installation. Installation planning and practices inside buildings.* London: BSI.

BSI (2020). PD CLC/TR 50174-99-2:2020 *Information technology. Cabling installation. Mitigation and protection from electrical interference.* London: BSI.

knx.org/knx-en/for-professionals/get-started/index.php

https://cedia.net/education-events

IEEE (2010). IEEE 1901-2010 *Standard for Broadband over Power Line Networks.* New York: IEEE.

IET (2016). *Code of Practice for Connected Systems Integration in Buildings.* London: IET Codes & Guidance.

IET (2019). *Code of Practice for Building Automation and Control Systems.* London: IET Codes & Guidance.

Energy

BSI (2019). BS HD 60364-8-1:2019 *Low-voltage electrical installations. Functional aspects. Energy efficiency.* London: BSI.

BSI (2019). BS HD 60364-8-2:2011+A11:2019 *Low-voltage electrical installations. Prosumer's low-voltage electrical installations.* London: BSI.

Department for Energy, Business and Industrial Strategy (2017). *Clean Growth Strategy.* [pdf] (Last updated 16 April 2018). Available at: https://www.gov.uk/government/publications/clean-growth-strategy

> *The Clean Growth Strategy identifies the key enablers and requirements of the shift to low-carbon transport and a low-carbon economy*

Appendix C – Suggested further reading and resources

EU Publications Office (2010). *Directive 2010/31/EU of the European Parliament and of the Council of 19 May 2010 on the energy performance of buildings (EPBD)*. [online] (Last reviewed 8 August 2018). Available at: https://eur-lex.europa.eu/legal-content/EN/ALL/;ELX_SESSIONID=FZMjThLLzfxmmMCQG p2Y1s2d3TjwtD8QS3pqdkhXZbwqGwlgY9KN!2064651424?uri=CELEX:32010L0031

https://energysavingtrust.org.uk/

https://www.gov.uk/guidance/domestic-private-rented-property-minimum-energy-efficiency-standard-landlord-guidance

IET (2015). *Code of Practice for Low and Extra Low Voltage Direct Current Power Distribution in Buildings*. London: IET Codes & Guidance.

IET (2017). *Code of Practice for Electrical Energy Storage Systems*. London: IET Codes & Guidance.

IET (2017). *Guide to Energy Management in the Built Environment*. London: IET Codes & Guidance.

Ministry of Housing, Communities & Local Government (2014). Approved Document L1A: *conservation of fuel and power in new dwellings*. [pdf] (Last updated 5 April 2018). Available at: https://www.gov.uk/government/publications/conservation-of-fuel-and-power-approved-document-l

EMC earthing and bonding

BSI (2016). BS EN 50310:2016+A1:2020 *Telecommunications bonding networks for buildings and other structures*. London: BSI.

BSI (2017). 17/30370687 DC: BS EN 60364-5-54 AMD1 *Low-voltage electrical installations. Part 5-54. Selection and erection of electrical equipment. Earthing arrangements and protective conductors*. London: BSI.

IET (2018). *Guidance Note 8: Earthing & Bonding*. 4th Edition. London: IET Codes & Guidance.

Cyber security

Department for Digital, Culture, Media & Sport (2019). *Secure by Design: The Government's Code of Practice for Consumer Internet of Things (IoT) Security for manufacturers, with guidance for consumers on smart devices at home*. [online] (Last updated: 6 June 2019). Available at: https://www.gov.uk/government/collections/secure-by-design

Information Commissioner's Office (2018). *Guide to the General Data Protection Regulation (GDPR)*. [online] (Last updated: January 2020). Available at: https://ico.org.uk/for-organisations/guide-to-data-protection/guide-to-the-general-data-protection-regulation-gdpr/

Assisted living

https://www.agileageing.org/

NHBC Foundation (2017). *Multigenerational living: an opportunity for UK house builders?*. [pdf] Available at: https://www.nhbcfoundation.org/publication/multigenerational-living-an-opportunity-for-uk-house-builders/

Electrotechnical reference

BEAMA (2018). *BEAMA Guide to Surge Protection Devices (SPDs) – Selection, Application and Theory*. [pdf] Available at: https://www.beama.org.uk/resourceLibrary/beama-surge-protection-guide-.html

Appendix C – Suggested further reading and resources

BEAMA (2019). *BEAMA Guide to Arc Fault Detection Devices (AFDDs)*. [pdf] Available at:
https://www.beama.org.uk/resourceLibrary/beama-guide-to-arc-fault-detection-devices--afdds.html

BEAMA (2019). *The RCD Handbook – Guide to the Selection and Application of Residual Current Devices (RCDs)*. [pdf] Available at: https://www.beama.org.uk/resourceLibrary/the-rcd-handbook---guide-to-the-selection-and-application-of-residual-current-devices.html

BSI (2018). BS 7671:2018+A1:2020 *Requirements for Electrical Installations. IET Wiring Regulations*. London: BSI.

IET (2014). *Code of Practice for the Application of LED Lighting Systems*. London: IET Codes & Guidance.

Smart home vision

BEAMA (2017). *Electrification by design series*. [pdf] Available at:
https://www.beama.org.uk/resource-library/electrification-by-design-series.html

CEDIA (2017). *Smart Home Infrastructure Recommended Guidelines*. Available at:
https://cedia.net/product.aspx?ID=1189

NHBC (2013). *Designing homes for the 21st century: lessons for low energy design*. [pdf] Available at:
https://www.nhbcfoundation.org/publication/designing-homes-for-the-21st-century/

NHBC Foundation (2016). *The connected home: designing and building technology into today's new homes*. [pdf] Available at: https://www.nhbcfoundation.org/publication/the-connected-home/

NHBC Foundation (2018). *Futurology: the new home in 2050*. [pdf] Available at:
https://www.nhbcfoundation.org/publication/nf80-futurology-the-new-home-in-2050/

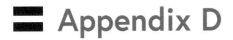 Appendix D

Templates

Smart home early contact template

Smart home guide early contact
Name:
Client address:
Installation address:
Starting when:
Deadline for finish:
New build, rewire or retrofit measure:
Size of installation:
Material: brick/block, timber frame, other:
Additional features on the property for connection:
QUESTIONS TO ASK THE CLIENT
How would you describe the character of the finished installation?
When will people be there?
Do you work from home?
What sort of functions or systems do you envisage in your smart home?
Who will be living in the home? Does anybody have any special needs?
What sort of things do you enjoy doing at home?
Is there anything I haven't asked about that you'd like me to consider?
Notes:

Appendix D – Templates

Consolidating needs template

Consolidating needs
Who is responsible for design?
Are plans available?
Who is responsible for project management? A builder?
List of non-portable electrical equipment to be connected:
List of systems the client would like to control:
List of things the client would like to be able to monitor:
List of rooms by name, with a summary of their use and an indication as to whether they might change use:
List of people who will occupy the home, including people who visit, e.g. cleaners/mobility team, children/grandchildren, parents/grandparents, pets:
Pattern of occupancy, daily, seasonally:
Does anyone in the home have any special needs?
Does anyone work from home?

Appendix D – Templates

Consolidating needs template (cont).

Is any later development planned?
Are there any events or circumstances that should be anticipated?
Is a change of occupancy or change of use likely?
What is the budget for the project? What is the budget for electrics?
Any other information that might affect the requirements of the house:

Appendix D – Templates

Functional analysis per-zone template

Functional analysis per-zone	
Project:	**Date:**
Zone:	**Room:**

Desired functions:
Luminaires:
Heating and cooling:
Motion sensing:
Touch controls:
Shading:
Audio/Visual:
Data:
Power:
Zone (repeat to confirm if loose pages used):
Other:
Notes:

Appendix D – Templates

Short-form functional analysis template

Short-form functional analysis
Client:
Install date:
Zone/Room:
Function:
Notes:

Appendix D – Templates

Method statement template

Project:	Activity:

Occurring when:

Operatives involved:

Description of activity:

Sketches:

Reference resources:

Training required:
Are outsourced specialists required?

Novel equipment/materials required:

Risk assessment carried out?

Actions required:

Method statement carried out by:

Version:

Appendix D – Templates

Smart home operational safety/safety-critical element template

Project:	
Smart home element:	
Risk:	
Risk mitigation:	

Designed by:	**Version:**	
Tested by:	**Date:**	

Appendix D – Templates

Bill of materials (BOM) template

Item	Item spec/link	Quantity	Cost exc.	Cost inc.	VAT	Credit terms	Purchase when	Supplier	Install phase 1-5	Lead time (days)	Note

Appendix D – Templates

Cable schedule template

Cable Schedule – Installation: **Version:**

Project:

Cable/size	To Zone/Room	Cable number	Description	Energy class	System	Emergence	Wire back to	Termination	Notes

Appendix D – Templates

Design audit template

Device	Input or output	Model	Energy	Power (W)	Likely cable	Bandwidth requirement	Number of cores required	SHHE connection type	Number required	Note

© The Institution of Engineering and Technology

Appendix D – Templates

Template for recording final circuits downstream of an MCB

Protective device	Location	Neutral termination	Line termination	Intermediate terminations	Module termination	Final circuits

Appendix D – Templates

MCB to final circuit schedule PER BREAKER template

Protection
6 A RCBO Type B

Location
DB1 (Upper) way 4

Circuits	Final cable ID			Module			I/O specifier		Note	

Appendix D – Templates

Example of how a functional analysis per-zone template can be adapted for use on handover

Project:	Date:	
Zone:	Room:	
Desired functions:		**Witnessed complete:**
Luminaires:		

Index

Index

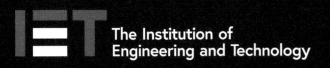

The Institution of Engineering and Technology

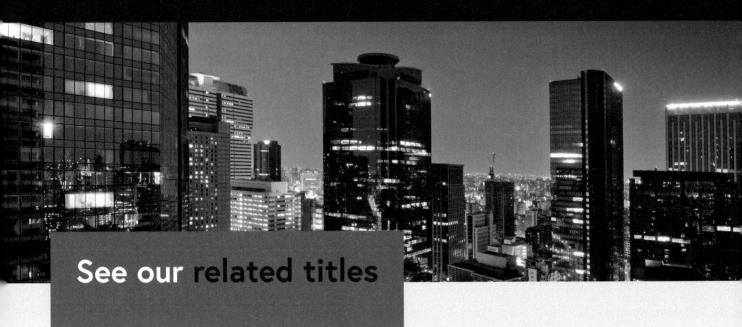

See our related titles

Smart home technologies often interact with multiple systems that each have their own, unique requirements for installation and maintenance. We have created guidance to address some of these systems directly, providing best-practice advice for installers and operators working with different electrical systems.

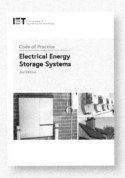

Code of Practice for Electrical Energy Storage Systems, 2nd Edition

This Code of Practice is an excellent reference for practitioners on the safe, effective and competent application of electrical energy storage systems. It provides detailed information on the specification, design, installation, commissioning, operation and maintenance of an electrical energy storage system.

Find out more: theiet.org/eess-mp

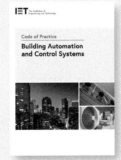

Code of Practice for Building Automation and Control Systems

This Code of Practice provides knowledge, understanding and good practice guidance on the design, evaluation and implementation of automated controls used in mechanical and electrical engineering systems within the built environment.

Find out more: theiet.org/bacs-mp

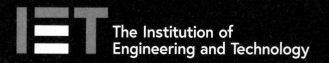

**The Institution of
Engineering and Technology**

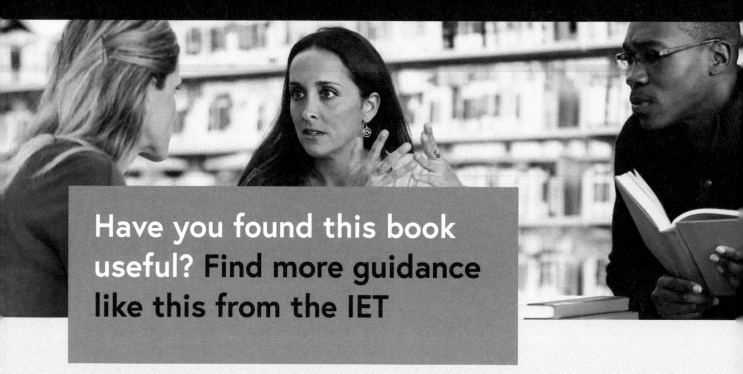

Have you found this book useful? Find more guidance like this from the IET

We bring together experts from across industry, providing practical guidance to help solve engineering problems in the real world.

Our Codes of Practice and guides are designed to advise on good practice across different areas of engineering, covering new and emerging technologies, and providing a consensus on specific challenges faced by engineers.

Topics include:

- Energy and renewables
- Building management and maintenance
- Electric vehicles
- Electrical safety
- Cyber security
- Healthcare

See our range of titles:
theiet.org./standards-books-mp

You can influence future standards like this in your field. See how you can get involved in the process at theiet.org/standards-involved-mp

The Institution of Engineering and Technology (IET) is registered as a Charity in England and Wales (No. 211014) and Scotland (No. SC038698).
The Institution of Engineering and Technology, Michael Faraday House, Six Hills Way, Stevenage, Hertfordshire SG1 2AY, United Kingdom.

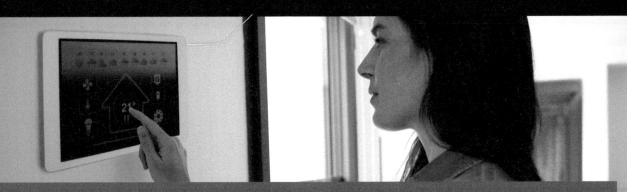

IET The Institution of Engineering and Technology

Academy

Complement your learning with 10% off* our online course: Smart Homes for Electrical Installers

Written by the author of this Guide, our e-learning course introduces the key principles and technologies involved in smart homes and describes some basic forms that smart homes can take.

This course will help you to:
- demonstrate a broad understanding of smart devices and smart measures within the built environment
- conduct a client and environment specific assessment of requirement encompassing smart technology
- create a viable technical specification and project plan for a smart home or smart measure
- create and execute a Construction Phase Plan encompassing smart measures
- manage an effective commissioning and client handover of a completed smart home
- offer appropriate technical support to the smart installation
- take reasonable measures to safeguard cyber security.

E-learning lets you study anytime, anywhere, with flexible access to expert content designed to help embed your learning through a variety of interactive training methods.

Find out more at **theiet.org/academy-about**

To claim your **10% discount***, visit theiet.org/academy-sh and enter code SHGuide10 at checkout.

Multi-user access for your business is available. See theiet.org/academy-business for details.

NOTES